THE VEGAN LOW FODMAP COOKBOOK

By

Jane F Garraway

Copyright © 2024

TABLE OF CONTENT

Navigating the Low-FODMAP Journey with Monash University

We have meticulously crafted every recipe in this cookbook to align with the low-FODMAP guidelines established by Monash University, the leading authority on the low-FODMAP diet. Monash University's pioneering research provides invaluable insights into which foods are suitable for individuals with irritable bowel syndrome (IBS) and other gastrointestinal sensitivities.

By relying on Monash University's comprehensive low-FODMAP food database, we've carefully curated ingredients that are low in fermentable carbohydrates and well-tolerated by those with digestive sensitivities. Our goal is to ensure that each recipe promotes digestive health, reduces discomfort, and delivers flavor-packed, nutritious meals.

Feel confident exploring these dishes, knowing they meet the latest low-FODMAP recommendations from Monash University. Your journey toward improved digestive well-being starts here—happy cooking and enjoy the flavorful path to relief!

The Low-FODMAP Diet: A Path to Digestive Wellness

The Low-FODMAP Diet offers tremendous benefits, helping individuals manage gastrointestinal distress while still enjoying delicious meals. Let's break down what the Low-FODMAP Diet is, how it works, and how to incorporate it into your life.

What is the Low-FODMAP Diet?

The Low-FODMAP Diet is a scientifically backed approach designed to limit certain carbohydrates and sugar alcohols known as Fermentable Oligosaccharides, Disaccharides, Monosaccharides, and Polyols (FODMAPs). These compounds can trigger bloating, gas, abdominal pain, and other digestive issues, particularly in individuals with IBS. The diet helps identify and manage these triggers, so you can enjoy a wide variety of foods without discomfort.

The Incredible Benefits of the Low-FODMAP Diet

- **Relief from Digestive Distress:** Reducing high-FODMAP foods can provide significant relief from symptoms like bloating and gas, allowing you to regain control over your digestive health.

- **Improved Gut Health:** Following the Low-FODMAP Diet gives your digestive system a chance to heal and function optimally, improving nutrient absorption and overall well-being.

- **Personalized Nutrition:** Everyone's tolerance to FODMAPs varies, and this diet helps you determine which foods work best for you.

- **Delicious Variety:** Despite the elimination of certain foods, the Low-FODMAP Diet offers a wide range of delicious and nutritious options, ensuring you don't feel deprived.

- **Enhanced Well-Being:** With fewer digestive issues, you'll likely experience higher energy levels, better mood, and an overall sense of wellness.

Implementing the Low-FODMAP Diet with Ease

Now that you understand the benefits, here's how to incorporate the Low-FODMAP Diet into your daily life:

1. **Consult a Professional:** Always seek advice from a registered dietitian or healthcare professional familiar with the Low-FODMAP Diet before making changes.

2. **Educate Yourself:** Learn about FODMAPs and their effects on the digestive system. Understanding these concepts will empower you to make informed decisions.

3. **Start with Elimination:** In the elimination phase, avoid high-FODMAP foods for a few weeks to pinpoint which ones trigger your symptoms.

4. **Keep a Food Diary:** Track your meals and any digestive symptoms. This will be helpful during consultations with healthcare professionals to tailor the diet to your specific needs.

5. **Reintroduce Foods Slowly:** After the elimination phase, gradually reintroduce FODMAP groups to test your tolerance. This will help you create a personalized diet that suits your unique digestive system.

6. **Explore Low-FODMAP Recipes:** Get creative in the kitchen with a variety of delicious low-FODMAP recipes. You'll be surprised at how enjoyable and satisfying the diet can be.

FODMAP Food List: Making Informed Choices for Digestive Health

Navigating the Low-FODMAP Diet can feel overwhelming at first, but with the right tools, it becomes manageable. This FODMAP Food List serves as a helpful guide to making informed choices. By understanding which foods are low in FODMAPs and which may trigger discomfort, you can confidently prepare meals that support digestive health.

Understanding FODMAPs

FODMAPs (Fermentable Oligosaccharides, Disaccharides, Monosaccharides, and Polyols) are types of carbohydrates and sugar alcohols that are poorly absorbed by the small intestine, causing discomfort for some people. The Low-FODMAP Diet is designed to minimize these foods, alleviating symptoms of bloating, gas, and pain.

Low-FODMAP Foods

Here's a list of commonly well-tolerated, low-FODMAP foods:

- **Fruits:** Bananas (ripe), blueberries, cantaloupe, grapes (up to 15), kiwi, oranges, pineapple, raspberries, strawberries

- **Vegetables:** Bell peppers (red, yellow), bok choy, carrots, cucumbers, green beans, lettuce, spinach, zucchini

- **Proteins:** Chicken, fish (salmon, cod, haddock), shrimp, firm tofu, turkey

- **Grains:** Quinoa, gluten-free oats, rice (white, basmati), cornmeal

- **Dairy & Alternatives:** Lactose-free milk and yogurt, hard cheeses (cheddar, Swiss), unsweetened almond milk, canned coconut milk

- **Nuts & Seeds:** Almonds (up to 10), chia seeds, macadamia nuts (up to 10), pumpkin seeds (up to 2 tbsp), sunflower seeds (up to 2 tbsp)

High-FODMAP Foods to Limit

These high-FODMAP foods may trigger digestive discomfort and should be avoided or consumed in limited amounts:

- **Fruits:** Apples, apricots, cherries, mangoes, pears, watermelon

- **Vegetables:** Artichokes, asparagus, cauliflower, garlic, onions, mushrooms

- **Proteins:** Beans (chickpeas, black beans, kidney beans), lentils, silken tofu, tempeh

- **Grains:** Wheat (bread, pasta), barley, rye, couscous

- **Dairy & Alternatives:** Cow's milk, soft cheeses (cottage cheese, ricotta), ice cream, soy milk

- **Nuts & Seeds:** Cashews, pistachios, peanuts

Remember that FODMAP sensitivity varies between individuals. Some people can tolerate small amounts of high-FODMAP foods, while others may need to eliminate them entirely. Use the elimination and reintroduction phases to personalize the diet to your digestive needs. Always consult with a dietitian to ensure you're meeting your nutritional requirements while following the Low-FODMAP Diet.

With this comprehensive FODMAP food guide, you can create satisfying, gut-friendly meals that suit your individual needs. The Low-FODMAP Diet is a powerful tool for identifying trigger foods and developing a long-term dietary plan that supports digestive comfort. Enjoy the journey to better gut health, and remember, you're not alone—professional guidance and community support are always available.

BREAKFASTS &

SMOOTHIES

French Toast

This recipe uses a low-FODMAP bread. You can use gluten-free or sourdough options.

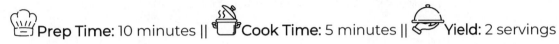 **Prep Time:** 10 minutes || **Cook Time:** 5 minutes || **Yield:** 2 servings

INGREDIENTS

- 2 slices low-FODMAP bread

- 1/2 cup unsweetened almond milk

- 1 tablespoon maple syrup

- 1 teaspoon vanilla extract

- 1/4 teaspoon cinnamon

- Coconut oil, for cooking

INSTRUCTIONS

1. In a shallow dish, whisk together almond milk, maple syrup, vanilla extract, and cinnamon.

2. Dip bread slices into the mixture, soaking both sides.

3. Heat coconut oil in a skillet over medium heat.

4. Cook the soaked bread slices until golden brown on both sides.

5. Serve with your favorite low-FODMAP toppings, such as maple syrup, fresh berries, or sugar-free syrup.

NOTES

- For a thicker french toast, increase the soaking time.

- You can experiment with different plant-based milk alternatives.

- Serve with a side of low-FODMAP bacon or sausage for a complete breakfast.

NUTRITIONAL INFORMATION (approximate per serving):

- Calories: 200 | Protein: 3g | Fat: 5g | Carbohydrates: 25g | Fiber: 2g | Sugar: 5g

Hash Browns

A classic breakfast side, adapted for a low-FODMAP diet. These crispy hash browns are packed with flavor and perfect for any meal.

Prep Time: 15 minutes || **Cook Time:** 20-25 minutes || **Yield:** 4 servings

INGREDIENTS

- 2 large potatoes, peeled and grated

- 1/4 onion, grated

- 1 tablespoon olive oil

- Salt and pepper to taste

INSTRUCTIONS

1. Place grated potatoes and onion in a clean kitchen towel or cheesecloth. Squeeze out as much excess moisture as possible.

2. Heat olive oil in a large skillet over medium heat.

3. Add the squeezed potato mixture to the skillet and spread it evenly.

4. Cook undisturbed for 5-7 minutes, or until golden brown and crispy on the bottom.

5. Carefully flip the hash browns and cook for another 5-7 minutes, or until golden brown and crispy on the other side.

6. Season with salt and pepper to taste. Serve immediately.

NOTES

- For extra crispy hash browns, let the potatoes air dry on a paper towel before squeezing out the moisture.

- You can add other grated vegetables, such as carrots or zucchini, for additional flavor and nutrients.

- Serve with your favorite low-FODMAP toppings, such as avocado, salsa, or vegan sour cream.

NUTRITIONAL INFORMATION (approximate per serving):

- Calories: 150 | Protein: 2g | Fat: 8g | Carbohydrates: 20g | Fiber: 2g | Sugar: 1g

Breakfast Hash

A hearty and satisfying breakfast or brunch option. Packed with vegetables and flavor, this hash is a great way to start your day.

Prep Time: 15 minutes || **Cook Time:** 20-25 minutes || **Yield:** 4 servings

INGREDIENTS

- 2 large potatoes, peeled and diced

- 1 red bell pepper, diced

- 1/2 onion, diced

- 1/4 cup frozen peas (thawed)

- 1 tablespoon olive oil

- 1/2 teaspoon paprika

- 1/4 teaspoon cumin

- Salt and pepper to taste

INSTRUCTIONS

1. Preheat a large skillet over medium heat.

2. Add olive oil to the skillet and then add potatoes, red bell pepper, and onion. Cook until softened and slightly browned, about 15 minutes.

3. Stir in thawed peas, paprika, cumin, salt, and pepper. Cook for an additional 2-3 minutes.

4. Serve hot with your favorite low-FODMAP toppings, such as avocado, salsa, or a fried egg (if not vegan).

NOTES

- For a spicier hash, add a pinch of cayenne pepper.

- You can add other vegetables to this hash, such as zucchini or mushrooms.

- Serve over a bed of greens for a lighter meal.

NUTRITIONAL INFORMATION (approximate per serving):

- Calories: 200 | Protein: 4g | Fat: 10g | Carbohydrates: 25g | Fiber: 3g | Sugar: 3g

Thai Green Curry

A fragrant and flavorful curry packed with vegetables. This low-FODMAP version is a satisfying and healthy meal.

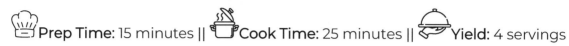

Prep Time: 15 minutes || **Cook Time:** 25 minutes || **Yield:** 4 servings

INGREDIENTS

- 1 tablespoon olive oil

- 1 onion, finely chopped

- 1 red bell pepper, sliced

- 1 green bell pepper, sliced

- 1 can (400g) light coconut milk

- 1 teaspoon green curry paste (low-FODMAP or homemade)

- 1 teaspoon red curry paste (low-FODMAP or homemade)

- 1 teaspoon fish sauce (gluten-free, low-FODMAP)

- 1 lime, juiced

- 1/2 teaspoon kaffir lime leaves (dried)

- Salt and pepper to taste

INSTRUCTIONS

1. Heat olive oil in a large pot or wok over medium heat. Add onion and cook until softened, about 5 minutes.

2. Stir in red and green bell peppers and cook for 5 minutes, or until slightly softened.

3. Add green curry paste and red curry paste to the pot. Cook for 1 minute, stirring constantly.

4. Pour in coconut milk and bring to a simmer. Add fish sauce, lime juice, and kaffir lime leaves. Season with salt and pepper.

5. Simmer for 15-20 minutes, or until the vegetables are tender.

6. Serve hot with brown rice or cauliflower rice.

NOTES

- For a thicker curry, reduce the cooking time or add a cornstarch slurry.

- You can add other low-FODMAP vegetables, such as zucchini or bamboo shoots, to the curry. Serve with a side of jasmine rice (low-FODMAP) for a complete meal.

NUTRITIONAL INFORMATION (approximate per serving):

- Calories: 300 | Protein: 5g | Fat: 15g | Carbohydrates: 25g | Fiber: 4g | Sugar: 5g

Tempeh Kimbab

Tempeh kimbab, a Korean-inspired roll, is a satisfying and nutritious meal. This low-FODMAP version is packed with flavor and perfect for meal prep. Kimbap traditionally uses seaweed sheets, but for this recipe, we'll use low-FODMAP rice paper sheets as a substitute.

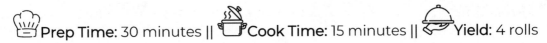 **Prep Time:** 30 minutes || **Cook Time:** 15 minutes || **Yield:** 4 rolls

INGREDIENTS

- 1 block tempeh, crumbled and marinated in low-FODMAP soy sauce and garlic powder

- 1 cup cooked brown rice (low-FODMAP)

- 1/2 cucumber, julienned

- 1 carrot, julienned

- 1 avocado, sliced

- 4 sheets rice paper

- Sesame seeds, for sprinkling

INSTRUCTIONS

1. Prepare the tempeh according to your preferred method (grilled, baked, or pan-fried).

2. Prepare the rice and let it cool completely.

3. Lay a rice paper sheet on a damp kitchen towel.

4. Spread a thin layer of cooked rice evenly over the rice paper, leaving a small margin at the edges.

5. Arrange tempeh, cucumber, carrot, and avocado slices in a line down the center of the rice.

6. Carefully roll up the rice paper, pressing firmly to seal.

7. Sprinkle with sesame seeds. Repeat with the remaining ingredients.

NOTES

- For additional flavor, you can add a thin layer of low-FODMAP mayonnaise or hummus before adding the fillings.

- Use a bamboo sushi rolling mat for easier rolling.

- Serve with low-FODMAP soy sauce or kimchi for dipping.

NUTRITIONAL INFORMATION (approximate per serving):

- Calories: 300 | Protein: 15g | Fat: 10g | Carbohydrates: 35g | Fiber: 4g | Sugar: 3g

Oatmeal Pancakes

Fluffy and flavorful pancakes that are gentle on the digestive system. These pancakes are packed with wholesome ingredients and perfect for a satisfying breakfast.

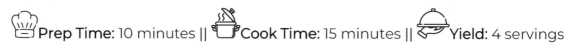

Prep Time: 10 minutes || **Cook Time:** 15 minutes || **Yield:** 4 servings

INGREDIENTS

- 1 cup gluten-free rolled oats

- 1/2 cup unsweetened almond milk (or other low-FODMAP milk)

- 1 ripe banana, mashed

- 1 tablespoon ground flaxseed mixed with 3 tablespoons water (flax egg)

- 1 teaspoon baking powder

- 1/4 teaspoon cinnamon

- Pinch of salt

- Optional toppings: maple syrup, fresh berries, coconut yogurt

INSTRUCTIONS

1. In a blender or food processor, combine oats, almond milk, mashed banana, flax egg, baking powder, cinnamon, and salt. Blend until smooth.

2. Heat a lightly oiled skillet or griddle over medium heat.

3. Pour 1/4 cup of batter onto the hot skillet for each pancake. Cook until bubbles form on the surface, then flip and cook until golden brown.

4. Serve immediately with your favorite low-FODMAP toppings.

NOTES

- For a thicker batter, add more oats or reduce the amount of almond milk.

- Experiment with different flavorings like vanilla extract or cardamon.

- To make these pancakes gluten-free, ensure the oats are certified gluten-free.

- For a nut-free option, use a different plant-based milk and omit any nut-based toppings.

NUTRITIONAL INFORMATION (approximate per serving):

- Calories: 200 | Protein: 7g | Fat: 5g | Carbohydrates: 30g | Fiber: 4g | Sugar: 10g

Dairy-Free Quiche

This recipe requires a low-FODMAP pie crust. You can purchase one or make your own using a low-FODMAP flour blend.

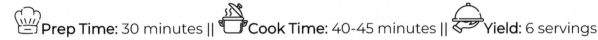 **Prep Time:** 30 minutes || **Cook Time:** 40-45 minutes || **Yield:** 6 servings

INGREDIENTS

For the filling:

- 1 block extra-firm tofu, pressed and crumbled

- 1/2 cup unsweetened almond milk

- 1/4 cup nutritional yeast

- 1 tablespoon lemon juice

- 1 teaspoon Dijon mustard

- 1/4 teaspoon garlic powder (optional)

- Salt and pepper to taste

- 1 cup spinach, chopped

- 1/2 cup cherry tomatoes, halved

INSTRUCTIONS

1. Preheat oven to 375°F (190°C).

2. In a large bowl, combine tofu, almond milk, nutritional yeast, lemon juice, Dijon mustard, garlic powder, salt, and pepper. Blend until smooth using an immersion blender or food processor.

3. Stir in spinach and cherry tomatoes.

4. Pour the filling into a prepared low-FODMAP pie crust.

5. Bake for 40-45 minutes, or until the filling is set.

6. Let cool slightly before serving.

NOTES

- For a richer filling, use full-fat coconut milk instead of almond milk.

- You can add other low-FODMAP vegetables to the filling, such as mushrooms or zucchini.

- Serve with a side salad or crusty bread for a complete meal.

NUTRITIONAL INFORMATION (approximate per serving):

- Calories: 200 | Protein: 10g | Fat: 10g | Carbohydrates: 20g | Fiber: 2g | Sugar: 3g

Chipotle Home Fries

A flavorful and satisfying breakfast or side dish. These crispy home fries are packed with smoky chipotle flavor and are completely free of high-FODMAP ingredients.

Prep Time: 10 minutes || **Cook Time:** 25-30 minutes || **Yield:** 4 servings

INGREDIENTS

- 2 large potatoes, peeled and cubed
- 1 tablespoon olive oil
- 1/2 teaspoon smoked paprika
- 1/4 teaspoon chili powder
- 1/4 teaspoon ground cumin
- Pinch of cayenne pepper (optional)
- 1/4 teaspoon chipotle chili powder
- Salt and pepper to taste

INSTRUCTIONS

1. Preheat oven to 400°F (200°C). Line a baking sheet with parchment paper.

2. In a large bowl, combine potato cubes, olive oil, smoked paprika, chili powder, cumin, cayenne pepper (if using), chipotle chili powder, salt, and pepper. Toss to coat.

3. Spread the potato mixture in a single layer on the prepared baking sheet.

4. Bake for 25-30 minutes, or until potatoes are golden brown and crispy. Stir halfway through cooking for even cooking.

5. Serve hot as a breakfast side dish or as a topping for bowls.

NOTES

- For extra crispy home fries, let the potatoes air dry on a paper towel before baking.

- Adjust the spice level to your taste by adding more or less chili powder and cayenne pepper.

- Serve with avocado, salsa, or vegan sour cream for a complete meal.

NUTRITIONAL INFORMATION (approximate per serving):

- Calories: 150 | Protein: 3g | Fat: 7g | Carbohydrates: 20g | Fiber: 2g | Sugar: 1g

Warm Chia Pudding

A comforting and nourishing breakfast or snack. This warm chia pudding is a unique twist on the traditional cold version.

Prep Time: 5 minutes || **Cook Time:** 5 minutes || **Yield:** 1 serving

INGREDIENTS

- 2 tablespoons chia seeds

- 1/2 cup unsweetened almond milk

- 1/4 teaspoon cinnamon

- Pinch of nutmeg

- Maple syrup to taste

INSTRUCTIONS

1. In a small saucepan, combine chia seeds, almond milk, cinnamon, and nutmeg.

2. Heat the mixture over low heat, stirring constantly, until the chia seeds bloom and the pudding thickens, about 5 minutes.

3. Remove from heat and let cool slightly.

4. Sweeten with maple syrup to taste.

NOTES

- For a thicker pudding, use a slightly higher ratio of chia seeds to liquid.

- You can add other flavors like vanilla extract or cocoa powder.

- Serve warm or chilled, topped with fresh berries or a sprinkle of nuts (low-FODMAP).

NUTRITIONAL INFORMATION (approximate per serving):

- Calories: 150 | Protein: 3g | Fat: 5g | Carbohydrates: 20g | Fiber: 5g | Sugar: 5g

Vanilla Chia Pudding

A classic breakfast or snack option, this chia pudding is packed with nutrients and low in FODMAPs.

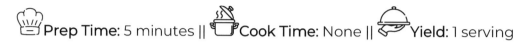 **Prep Time:** 5 minutes || **Cook Time:** None || **Yield:** 1 serving

INGREDIENTS

- 3 tablespoons chia seeds

- 1/2 cup unsweetened almond milk

- 1 teaspoon vanilla extract

- 1 tablespoon maple syrup (or to taste)

- Pinch of salt

INSTRUCTIONS

1. In a jar or bowl, combine chia seeds, almond milk, vanilla extract, maple syrup, and salt.

2. Stir well to ensure no clumps of chia seeds.

3. Cover and refrigerate for at least 2 hours, or overnight, allowing the chia seeds to fully hydrate and thicken the pudding.

4. Stir before serving and enjoy!

NOTES

- For a thicker pudding, use a slightly higher ratio of chia seeds to liquid.

- You can add other flavors like cocoa powder or fruit puree for variation.

- Top with fresh berries, nuts (low-FODMAP), or granola for added texture and flavor.

NUTRITIONAL INFORMATION (approximate per serving):

- Calories: 150 | Protein: 3g | Fat: 5g | Carbohydrates: 20g | Fiber: 5g | Sugar: 5g

Mixed Berry Smoothie

A refreshing and antioxidant-packed smoothie perfect for any time of day.

Prep Time: 5 minutes || **Cook Time:** None || **Yield:** 1 serving

INGREDIENTS

- 1/2 cup mixed berries (strawberries, raspberries, blueberries - low-FODMAP serving sizes)

- 1/2 cup unsweetened almond milk

- 1 tablespoon chia seeds

- 1/4 teaspoon vanilla extract

- Optional: a drizzle of honey or maple syrup (low-FODMAP)

INSTRUCTIONS

1. Combine all ingredients in a blender.

2. Blend until smooth and creamy.

3. Adjust sweetness to taste by adding a low-FODMAP sweetener if needed.

NOTES

- For a thicker smoothie, use frozen berries or add a handful of ice cubes.

- You can experiment with different low-FODMAP fruits for variety.

- Top with a sprinkle of chia seeds or a dollop of coconut yogurt for added texture.

NUTRITIONAL INFORMATION (approximate per serving):

- Calories: 150 | Protein: 3g | Fat: 5g | Carbohydrates: 25g | Fiber: 4g | Sugar: 10g

Sweet Potato Pancakes

These fluffy pancakes are packed with the natural sweetness of sweet potatoes and are perfect for a satisfying breakfast.

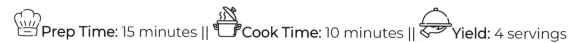

Prep Time: 15 minutes || **Cook Time:** 10 minutes || **Yield:** 4 servings

INGREDIENTS

- 1 large sweet potato, peeled and shredded

- 1/2 cup gluten-free oat flour

- 1 tablespoon ground flaxseed mixed with 3 tablespoons water (flax egg)

- 1 teaspoon baking powder

- Pinch of salt

- 1/4 cup unsweetened almond milk

- Maple syrup, for serving

- Optional toppings: fresh berries, sliced banana

INSTRUCTIONS

1. Preheat a large skillet over medium heat.

2. In a bowl, combine shredded sweet potato, oat flour, flax egg, baking powder, and salt.

3. Stir in almond milk until just combined.

4. Cook pancakes in the heated skillet, using about 1/4 cup of batter for each pancake. Cook until golden brown on both sides.

5. Serve immediately with maple syrup and your desired toppings.

NOTES

- For a thicker pancake, add more oat flour or reduce the amount of almond milk.

- You can add a pinch of cinnamon or nutmeg to the batter for extra flavor.

- Serve with a side of bacon or sausage (low-FODMAP options) for a complete breakfast.

NUTRITIONAL INFORMATION (approximate per serving):

- Calories: 200 | Protein: 5g | Fat: 5g | Carbohydrates: 30g | Fiber: 3g | Sugar: 5g

Matcha Overnight Oats

A refreshing and energizing breakfast packed with antioxidants. This creamy and satisfying oat-based treat is perfect for busy mornings.

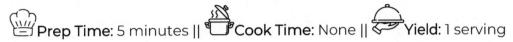**Prep Time:** 5 minutes || **Cook Time:** None || **Yield:** 1 serving

INGREDIENTS

- 1/2 cup gluten-free rolled oats

- 1/2 cup unsweetened almond milk (or other low-FODMAP milk)

- 1 tablespoon chia seeds

- 1 teaspoon matcha powder

- 1-2 teaspoons maple syrup (or to taste)

- Pinch of salt

- Optional toppings: fresh berries, sliced banana, a sprinkle of coconut flakes

INSTRUCTIONS

1. In a jar or bowl, combine oats, chia seeds, matcha powder, maple syrup, and salt.

2. Pour almond milk over the mixture. Stir well to combine.

3. Cover and refrigerate overnight.

4. In the morning, stir the oats again. Top with your desired toppings and enjoy.

NOTES

- For a thicker consistency, add more chia seeds or reduce the amount of almond milk.

- Experiment with different flavors by adding a splash of vanilla extract or a pinch of cinnamon.

- If you prefer a sweeter taste, you can increase the amount of maple syrup.

- Always check the labels of store-bought products to ensure they are low-FODMAP.

NUTRITIONAL INFORMATION (approximate per serving):

- Calories: 250 | Protein: 7g | Fat: 8g | Carbohydrates: 35g | Fiber: 5g | Sugar: 10g

Green Detox Smoothie

A refreshing and nutrient-packed smoothie to kickstart your day. This low-FODMAP version is packed with antioxidants and is gentle on the digestive system.

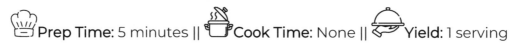

Prep Time: 5 minutes || **Cook Time:** None || **Yield:** 1 serving

INGREDIENTS

- 1 cup spinach or kale

- 1/2 cup pineapple (low-FODMAP serving size)

- 1/2 banana (or use a low-FODMAP sweetener)

- 1/2 cup unsweetened almond milk

- 1 tablespoon chia seeds

- 1 teaspoon lemon juice

- 1/2 teaspoon grated ginger

- Optional: a scoop of low-FODMAP protein powder

INSTRUCTIONS

1. Combine all ingredients in a blender.

2. Blend until smooth and creamy.

3. Adjust sweetness to taste by adding a low-FODMAP sweetener if needed.

NOTES

- For a thicker smoothie, add more spinach or kale.

- Experiment with different greens and fruits to vary the flavor.

- You can add a handful of ice cubes for a colder smoothie.

- For extra protein, use a low-FODMAP protein powder.

NUTRITIONAL INFORMATION (approximate per serving):

- Calories: 200 | Protein: 5g | Fat: 5g | Carbohydrates: 30g | Fiber: 5g | Sugar: 10g

Tropical Smoothie Bowl

A refreshing and vibrant breakfast or snack, this smoothie bowl is packed with tropical flavors.

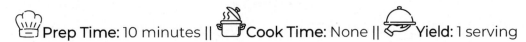 **Prep Time:** 10 minutes || **Cook Time:** None || **Yield:** 1 serving

INGREDIENTS

- 1/2 cup frozen pineapple chunks (low-FODMAP serving size)
- 1/2 cup frozen mango chunks (low-FODMAP serving size)
- 1/4 cup unsweetened coconut milk
- 1 tablespoon chia seeds
- 1/4 teaspoon vanilla extract
- Optional toppings: fresh fruit, granola, coconut flakes, nuts (low-FODMAP)

INSTRUCTIONS

1. Combine frozen pineapple, frozen mango, coconut milk, chia seeds, and vanilla extract in a blender.
2. Blend until smooth and creamy.
3. Pour the smoothie base into a bowl.
4. Top with your desired toppings.

NOTES

- For a thicker smoothie, use less liquid or add frozen banana (in moderation).
- Adjust sweetness by adding a low-FODMAP sweetener if needed.
- Experiment with different tropical fruits like papaya or passionfruit.

NUTRITIONAL INFORMATION (approximate per serving):

- Calories: 200 | Protein: 3g | Fat: 5g | Carbohydrates: 30g | Fiber: 5g | Sugar: 15g

Ginger and Pear Smoothie

A comforting and warming smoothie perfect for colder days. This low-FODMAP blend offers a unique flavor combination.

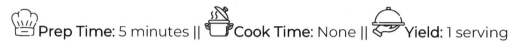

Prep Time: 5 minutes || **Cook Time:** None || **Yield:** 1 serving

INGREDIENTS

- 1/2 pear, peeled and chopped

- 1/2 cup unsweetened almond milk

- 1 teaspoon grated ginger

- 1 tablespoon chia seeds

- 1/4 teaspoon cinnamon

- Optional: a drizzle of honey or maple syrup (low-FODMAP)

INSTRUCTIONS

1. Combine all ingredients in a blender.

2. Blend until smooth and creamy.

3. Adjust sweetness to taste by adding a low-FODMAP sweetener if needed.

NOTES

- For a thicker smoothie, use frozen pear or add a handful of ice cubes.

- You can add a squeeze of lemon juice for a tangy twist.

- Garnish with a sprinkle of cinnamon or grated ginger for presentation.

NUTRITIONAL INFORMATION (approximate per serving):

- Calories: 150 | Protein: 3g | Fat: 5g | Carbohydrates: 25g | Fiber: 4g | Sugar: 10g

Blueberry Breakfast Quinoa

A healthy and satisfying breakfast option, this quinoa dish is packed with antioxidants and fiber.

Prep Time: 10 minutes || **Cook Time:** 15 minutes || **Yield:** 1 serving

INGREDIENTS

- 1/2 cup quinoa, rinsed

- 1 cup unsweetened almond milk

- 1/2 cup blueberries (low-FODMAP serving size)

- 1 tablespoon chia seeds

- 1 teaspoon maple syrup

- 1/4 teaspoon cinnamon

- Pinch of salt

INSTRUCTIONS

1. In a small saucepan, combine quinoa and almond milk. Bring to a boil, then reduce heat, cover, and simmer for 15 minutes, or until quinoa is fluffy.

2. Stir in blueberries, chia seeds, maple syrup, cinnamon, and salt.

3. Let cool for a few minutes before serving.

NOTES

- For a thicker pudding-like texture, let the quinoa cool completely before serving.

- You can add other low-FODMAP fruits or nuts for variation.

- Serve warm or cold, depending on your preference.

NUTRITIONAL INFORMATION (approximate per serving):

- Calories: 200 | Protein: 5g | Fat: 3g | Carbohydrates: 35g | Fiber: 5g | Sugar: 10g

Carrot Strawberry Smoothie

A refreshing and nutritious smoothie packed with vitamins and antioxidants. This low-FODMAP version is a perfect way to start your day.

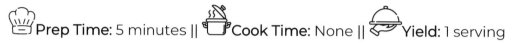**Prep Time:** 5 minutes || **Cook Time:** None || **Yield:** 1 serving

INGREDIENTS

- 1/2 cup chopped carrots

- 1/2 cup fresh strawberries (low-FODMAP serving size)

- 1/2 cup unsweetened almond milk

- 1 tablespoon chia seeds

- 1 teaspoon lemon juice

- Optional: a scoop of low-FODMAP protein powder

INSTRUCTIONS

1. Combine all ingredients in a blender.

2. Blend until smooth and creamy.

3. Adjust sweetness to taste by adding a low-FODMAP sweetener if needed.

NOTES

- For a sweeter smoothie, add a ripe banana (in moderation).

- You can add a handful of ice cubes for a colder smoothie.

- Experiment with different low-FODMAP fruits and vegetables for variety.

NUTRITIONAL INFORMATION (approximate per serving):

- Calories: 150 | Protein: 3g | Fat: 5g | Carbohydrates: 25g | Fiber: 4g | Sugar: 10g

Matcha and Mango Smoothie

A refreshing and energizing blend of matcha and mango. This low-FODMAP smoothie is packed with antioxidants and provides a natural energy boost.

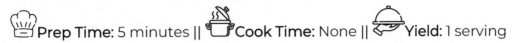 **Prep Time:** 5 minutes || **Cook Time:** None || **Yield:** 1 serving

INGREDIENTS

- 1/2 ripe mango, chopped

- 1/2 cup unsweetened almond milk

- 1 teaspoon matcha powder

- 1 tablespoon chia seeds

- 1/2 teaspoon lemon juice

- Optional: a drizzle of honey or maple syrup (low-FODMAP)

INSTRUCTIONS

1. Combine all ingredients in a blender.

2. Blend until smooth and creamy.

3. Adjust sweetness to taste by adding a low-FODMAP sweetener if needed.

NOTES

- For a thicker smoothie, use frozen mango or add a handful of ice cubes.

- You can experiment with different plant-based milk alternatives.

- Garnish with a sprinkle of matcha powder or a slice of mango for presentation.

NUTRITIONAL INFORMATION (approximate per serving):

- Calories: 150 | Protein: 3g | Fat: 5g | Carbohydrates: 25g | Fiber: 4g | Sugar: 10g

Note: This recipe is a general guide. Always consult with a healthcare professional or registered dietitian for personalized dietary advice.

Banana Bread Baked Steel Cut Oats

This hearty and comforting dish combines the best of both worlds: the wholesome goodness of steel cut oats and the indulgent flavors of banana bread.

Prep Time: 15 minutes || **Cook Time:** 45-50 minutes || **Yield:** 6 servings

INGREDIENTS

- 1 cup steel cut oats

- 2 ripe bananas, mashed

- 1/2 cup unsweetened almond milk

- 1/4 cup maple syrup

- 1 teaspoon vanilla extract

- 1 teaspoon baking powder

- 1/2 teaspoon cinnamon

- Pinch of salt

- Optional: chopped walnuts or pecans (check for low-FODMAP serving sizes)

INSTRUCTIONS

1. Preheat oven to 350°F (175°C). Grease a baking dish.

2. In a large bowl, combine mashed bananas, almond milk, maple syrup, and vanilla extract.

3. Stir in steel cut oats, baking powder, cinnamon, and salt.

4. Optional: Fold in chopped nuts.

5. Pour the mixture into the prepared baking dish.

6. Bake for 45-50 minutes, or until golden brown and set.

7. Let cool slightly before serving.

NOTES

- For a richer flavor, add a tablespoon of coconut oil or nut butter to the batter.

- Top with fresh berries or a drizzle of maple syrup for extra sweetness.

- This dish can be prepared ahead of time and reheated for a quick breakfast.

NUTRITIONAL INFORMATION (approximate per serving):

- Calories: 250 | Protein: 6g | Fat: 5g | Carbohydrates: 40g | Fiber: 4g | Sugar: 10g

Quinoa Porridge with Berries and Cinnamon

A warm and comforting breakfast that's packed with nutrients. This low-FODMAP quinoa porridge is quick and easy to make, and perfect for starting your day.

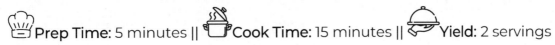 **Prep Time:** 5 minutes || **Cook Time:** 15 minutes || **Yield:** 2 servings

INGREDIENTS

- 1/2 cup quinoa, rinsed

- 1 cup unsweetened almond milk

- 1/4 teaspoon cinnamon

- Pinch of salt

- Maple syrup (to taste)

- Fresh or frozen mixed berries

- Optional toppings: sliced almonds, chia seeds

INSTRUCTIONS

1. In a medium saucepan, combine quinoa, almond milk, cinnamon, and salt.

2. Bring to a boil, then reduce heat to low, cover, and simmer for 15 minutes, or until quinoa is tender and liquid is absorbed.

3. Stir occasionally to prevent sticking.

4. Remove from heat and let cool slightly.

5. Serve warm topped with fresh or frozen mixed berries, maple syrup, and optional toppings like sliced almonds or chia seeds.

NOTES

- For a creamier porridge, use a blender to puree the cooked quinoa.

- Adjust sweetness to taste by adding more or less maple syrup.

- Experiment with different toppings like coconut flakes, chopped nuts, or a drizzle of nut butter.

- Store leftovers in the refrigerator for up to 3 days.

NUTRITIONAL INFORMATION (approximate per serving):

- Calories: 200 | Protein: 5g | Fat: 3g | Carbohydrates: 35g | Fiber: 3g | Sugar: 5g

LUNCH & DINNER

Potato Salad

A classic summer side dish, adapted for a low-FODMAP diet. This version is creamy and flavorful, without compromising on taste.

Prep Time: 20 minutes || **Cook Time:** 20 minutes || **Yield:** 4 servings

INGREDIENTS

- 1.5 lbs small, waxy potatoes

- 1/4 cup vegan mayonnaise (low-FODMAP)

- 2 tablespoons Dijon mustard

- 1 tablespoon white wine vinegar

- 1 teaspoon dried dill

- Salt and pepper to taste

- Optional: chopped celery, chopped chives

INSTRUCTIONS

1. Boil potatoes in salted water until tender, about 20 minutes. Drain and let cool completely.

2. Dice the cooled potatoes into bite-sized pieces.

3. In a large bowl, combine vegan mayonnaise, Dijon mustard, white wine vinegar, dill, salt, and pepper.

4. Gently fold the potatoes into the dressing, ensuring they are evenly coated.

5. Stir in chopped celery and chives, if using.

6. Refrigerate for at least 30 minutes before serving to allow flavors to meld.

NOTES

- For a richer flavor, use a combination of vegan mayonnaise and plain Greek-style yogurt.

- Adjust the acidity by adding more or less white wine vinegar.

- Serve chilled for a refreshing side dish.

NUTRITIONAL INFORMATION (approximate per serving):

- Calories: 200 | Protein: 3g | Fat: 10g | Carbohydrates: 25g | Fiber: 2g | Sugar: 2g

Tofu Teriyaki

A classic combination of flavors, adapted to be low-FODMAP. This tofu teriyaki is a quick and satisfying meal.

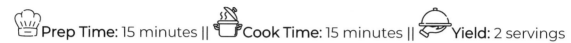 **Prep Time:** 15 minutes || **Cook Time:** 15 minutes || **Yield:** 2 servings

INGREDIENTS

For the Tofu:

- 1 block extra-firm tofu, pressed and cubed

- 2 tablespoons cornstarch

- 2 tablespoons low-sodium tamari

- 1 tablespoon sesame oil

For the Teriyaki Sauce:

- 1/4 cup low-sodium tamari

- 1 tablespoon rice vinegar

- 1 tablespoon maple syrup

- 1 teaspoon minced ginger

INSTRUCTIONS

1. Press the tofu to remove excess water. Cut into cubes. Combine cornstarch and tamari in a bowl. Toss tofu cubes in this mixture to coat.

2. Heat sesame oil in a skillet over medium heat. Cook tofu cubes until golden brown on all sides. Remove from skillet and set aside.

3. In a small bowl, whisk together tamari, rice vinegar, maple syrup, and ginger.

4. Return the tofu to the skillet and pour the teriyaki sauce over it. Cook for a few minutes until the sauce thickens and coats the tofu.

NOTES

- Serve with low-FODMAP sides like brown rice, zucchini noodles, or steamed broccoli.

- For a thicker sauce, you can add a cornstarch slurry (1 tablespoon cornstarch mixed with 2 tablespoons water).

- Adjust the sweetness of the teriyaki sauce by adding more or less maple syrup.

NUTRITIONAL INFORMATION (approximate per serving):

- Calories: 300 | Protein: 15g | Fat: 10g | Carbohydrates: 20g | Fiber: 2g | Sugar: 5g

Falafel

A crispy and flavorful Middle Eastern classic, adapted to be low-FODMAP. These falafel are packed with protein and perfect for a satisfying meal.

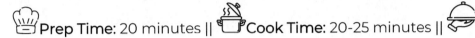 **Prep Time:** 20 minutes || **Cook Time:** 20-25 minutes || **Yield:** 4 servings

INGREDIENTS

- 1 can (15 oz) chickpeas, rinsed and drained

- 1/2 cup finely chopped parsley

- 1/4 cup finely chopped cilantro

- 1/4 cup finely chopped green onions

- 1 clove garlic, minced (optional, for those with mild FODMAP intolerance)

- 1/4 cup gluten-free oat flour

- 1 teaspoon ground cumin

- 1/2 teaspoon coriander

- 1/4 teaspoon baking powder

- Salt and pepper to taste

- Olive oil, for frying

INSTRUCTIONS

1. In a food processor, combine chickpeas, parsley, cilantro, green onions, garlic (if using), oat flour, cumin, coriander, baking powder, salt, and pepper. Pulse until mixture forms a thick paste.

2. Shape the mixture into small balls, about 1 inch in diameter.

3. Heat olive oil in a deep skillet over medium heat.

4. Fry falafel balls in batches until golden brown and crispy on all sides.

5. Remove falafel from the oil and drain on paper towels.

6. Serve hot with your favorite low-FODMAP toppings, such as hummus, tahini, or tzatziki sauce.

NOTES

- For a healthier option, bake the falafel in a preheated oven at 400°F (200°C) for 20-25 minutes, or until golden brown.

- Serve in pita bread (low-FODMAP) with your favorite fillings for a complete meal.

NUTRITIONAL INFORMATION (approximate per serving):

- Calories: 250 | Protein: 10g | Fat: 12g | Carbohydrates: 25g | Fiber: 5g | Sugar: 2g

Lentil Curry

A hearty and flavorful curry packed with protein and fiber. This low-FODMAP version is a comforting and satisfying meal.

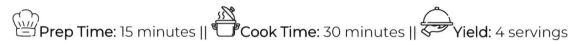 **Prep Time:** 15 minutes || **Cook Time:** 30 minutes || **Yield:** 4 servings

INGREDIENTS

- 1 tablespoon garlic-infused olive oil

- 1 onion, finely chopped

- 1 inch piece of ginger, grated

- 1 teaspoon ground cumin

- 1 teaspoon ground coriander

- 1/2 teaspoon turmeric

- 1/4 teaspoon red pepper flakes (optional)

- 1 can (400g) crushed tomatoes

- 1 can (400g) green lentils, rinsed and drained

- 400ml coconut milk

- Salt and pepper to taste

- Fresh cilantro, for garnish (optional)

- Optional: a squeeze of lime juice

INSTRUCTIONS

1. Heat olive oil in a large pot over medium heat. Add onion and ginger, cook until softened, about 5 minutes.

2. Stir in cumin, coriander, turmeric, and red pepper flakes. Cook for 30 seconds more.

3. Add crushed tomatoes, lentils, and coconut milk to the pot. Bring to a boil, then reduce heat and simmer for 20-25 minutes, or until lentils are tender.

4. Season with salt and pepper to taste.

5. Serve hot, garnished with fresh cilantro and a squeeze of lime juice (optional).

NOTES

- For a thicker curry, use less coconut milk or simmer for a longer period.

- Serve with brown rice or cauliflower rice for a complete meal.

- This curry can be made ahead of time and reheated.

NUTRITIONAL INFORMATION (approximate per serving):

- Calories: 350 | Protein: 15g | Fat: 15g | Carbohydrates: 30g | Fiber: 8g | Sugar: 5g

Lentil Daal

A hearty and comforting lentil daal, adapted for a low-FODMAP diet. This version is packed with flavor and protein.

Prep Time: 15 minutes || **Cook Time:** 30 minutes || **Yield:** 4 servings

INGREDIENTS

- 1 tablespoon olive oil
- 1 onion, finely chopped
- 1 inch ginger, grated
- 1 teaspoon cumin
- 1 teaspoon coriander
- 1/2 teaspoon turmeric

- 1/4 teaspoon red pepper flakes (optional)
- 1 can (400g) crushed tomatoes
- 1 can (400g) green lentils, rinsed and drained
- 400ml coconut milk
- Salt and pepper to taste
- Fresh cilantro, for garnish (optional)

INSTRUCTIONS

1. Heat olive oil in a large pot over medium heat. Add onion and ginger, cook until softened, about 5 minutes.

2. Stir in cumin, coriander, turmeric, and red pepper flakes. Cook for 30 seconds more.

3. Add crushed tomatoes, lentils, and coconut milk to the pot. Bring to a boil, then reduce heat and simmer for 20-25 minutes, or until lentils are tender.

4. Season with salt and pepper to taste.

5. Serve hot, garnished with fresh cilantro (optional).

NOTES

- For a thicker daal, simmer for a longer period or use less coconut milk.

- Serve with brown rice or cauliflower rice for a complete meal.

- This daal can be made ahead of time and reheated.

NUTRITIONAL INFORMATION (approximate per serving):

- Calories: 300 | Protein: 15g | Fat: 12g | Carbohydrates: 30g | Fiber: 6g | Sugar: 5g

Tofu Fried Rice

A classic comfort food with a low-FODMAP twist. This tofu fried rice is packed with flavor and perfect for a quick and easy meal.

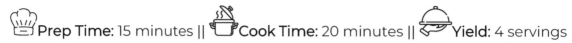 **Prep Time:** 15 minutes || **Cook Time:** 20 minutes || **Yield:** 4 servings

INGREDIENTS

- 1 block extra-firm tofu, pressed and cubed

- 2 cups cooked brown rice (low-FODMAP)

- 1 carrot, diced

- 1/2 cup frozen peas, thawed

- 2 green onions, thinly sliced

- 2 tablespoons soy sauce (low-sodium, tamari)

- 1 tablespoon sesame oil

- 1 teaspoon rice vinegar

- 1/2 teaspoon ginger powder

- Salt and pepper to taste

INSTRUCTIONS

1. Heat sesame oil in a large skillet over medium heat. Add tofu and cook until golden brown, about 5 minutes. Remove from skillet and set aside.

2. Add carrots and green onions to the skillet and cook for 2-3 minutes, or until softened.

3. Stir in cooked rice, soy sauce, rice vinegar, ginger powder, salt, and pepper. Cook for 5 minutes, or until heated through.

4. Return tofu to the skillet and combine well.

5. Stir in frozen peas and cook for an additional minute, or until heated through.

6. Serve immediately.

NOTES

- For added flavor, you can add a drizzle of sesame oil before serving.

- This recipe can be customized with your favorite low-FODMAP vegetables.

- Serve with a side of stir-fried bok choy or edamame for a complete meal.

NUTRITIONAL INFORMATION (approximate per serving):

- Calories: 300 | Protein: 15g | Fat: 10g | Carbohydrates: 40g | Fiber: 3g | Sugar: 2g

Pumpkin Soup

A creamy and comforting soup perfect for colder days. This low-FODMAP version is packed with flavor and gentle on the digestive system.

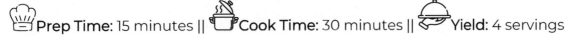 **Prep Time:** 15 minutes || **Cook Time:** 30 minutes || **Yield:** 4 servings

INGREDIENTS

- 1 tablespoon olive oil

- 1 onion, finely chopped

- 1 leek, white part only, finely chopped

- 1 clove garlic, minced (optional, for those with mild FODMAP intolerance)

- 1 inch piece of ginger, grated

- 1 teaspoon ground cumin

- 1/2 teaspoon ground coriander

- 1/4 teaspoon red pepper flakes (optional)

- 1 can (400g) pumpkin puree

- 4 cups vegetable broth

- 1/2 cup coconut milk

- Salt and pepper to taste

- Fresh sage or thyme, for garnish (optional)

INSTRUCTIONS

1. Heat olive oil in a large pot over medium heat. Add onion, leek, and garlic (if using), cook until softened, about 5 minutes.

2. Stir in ginger, cumin, coriander, and red pepper flakes. Cook for 30 seconds more.

3. Add pumpkin puree, vegetable broth, and coconut milk to the pot. Bring to a boil, then reduce heat and simmer for 15-20 minutes, or until heated through.

4. Season with salt and pepper to taste.

5. Puree the soup using an immersion blender or blender until smooth. Serve hot.

NOTES

- For a thicker soup, use less vegetable broth or add a cornstarch slurry.

- Serve with a dollop of vegan yogurt or a sprinkle of pumpkin seeds for added texture.

NUTRITIONAL INFORMATION (approximate per serving):

- Calories: 200 | Protein: 3g | Fat: 10g | Carbohydrates: 25g | Fiber: 3g | Sugar: 5g

Hummus Wrap

A refreshing and satisfying wrap packed with flavor and nutrients. This low-FODMAP option is perfect for a quick and healthy lunch or snack.

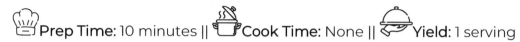 **Prep Time:** 10 minutes || **Cook Time:** None || **Yield:** 1 serving

INGREDIENTS

- 1 low-FODMAP tortilla (corn or gluten-free)

- 1/4 cup low-FODMAP hummus

- 2-3 leaves romaine lettuce, shredded

- 1/4 cup cucumber, sliced

- 1/4 cup red bell pepper, sliced

- 1 tablespoon grated carrot

- Optional: a sprinkle of fresh dill or parsley

INSTRUCTIONS

1. Lay out the tortilla flat on a clean surface.

2. Spread a layer of low-FODMAP hummus evenly over the tortilla.

3. Top with shredded romaine lettuce, cucumber slices, red bell pepper slices, and grated carrot.

4. Sprinkle with fresh dill or parsley, if desired.

5. Carefully roll up the tortilla to form a wrap.

NOTES

- Use your favorite low-FODMAP vegetables to customize your wrap.

- For extra flavor, add a drizzle of olive oil or a squeeze of lemon juice.

- To make this wrap ahead of time, prepare the ingredients and assemble the wraps just before eating for optimal freshness.

NUTRITIONAL INFORMATION (approximate per serving):

- Calories: 250 | Protein: 5g | Fat: 10g | Carbohydrates: 30g | Fiber: 4g | Sugar: 3g

Veggie Burger

A hearty and flavorful plant-based burger that's perfect for a satisfying meal. Packed with protein and low in FODMAPs, it's a delicious and healthy option.

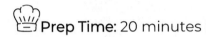**Prep Time:** 20 minutes || 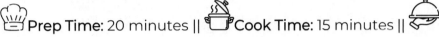**Cook Time:** 15 minutes || 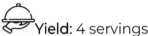**Yield:** 4 servings

INGREDIENTS

- 1 can (15 oz) chickpeas, rinsed and drained

- 1/2 cup cooked brown rice or quinoa

- 1/2 cup grated carrot

- 1/4 cup chopped onion

- 1/4 cup breadcrumbs (gluten-free and low-FODMAP)

- 1 tablespoon ground flaxseed mixed with 3 tablespoons water (flax egg)

- 1 teaspoon garlic powder (optional, for those with mild FODMAP intolerance)

- 1/2 teaspoon cumin

- 1/4 teaspoon paprika

- Salt and pepper to taste

INSTRUCTIONS

1. In a large bowl, mash chickpeas with a fork, leaving some whole chickpeas for texture.

2. Add cooked rice or quinoa, grated carrot, chopped onion, breadcrumbs, flax egg, garlic powder, cumin, paprika, salt, and pepper to the chickpeas. Mix well until combined.

3. Shape the mixture into four patties.

4. Heat a large skillet over medium heat with a drizzle of olive oil.

5. Cook patties for 5-7 minutes per side, or until golden brown and cooked through.

6. Serve on a low-FODMAP bun with your favorite toppings, such as lettuce, tomato, and vegan mayo.

NOTES

- To make the patties hold together better, refrigerate the mixture for 30 minutes before shaping.

- Serve with a side of sweet potato fries or a green salad for a complete meal.

NUTRITIONAL INFORMATION (approximate per serving):

- Calories: 250 | Protein: 15g | Fat: 5g | Carbohydrates: 30g | Fiber: 6g | Sugar: 3g

Veggie Stir Fry

A quick and easy stir-fry packed with colorful vegetables and savory flavors. This recipe is perfect for a healthy and satisfying meal that's gentle on the digestive system.

Prep Time: 15 minutes || **Cook Time:** 10-15 minutes || **Yield:** 2 servings

INGREDIENTS

- 1 tablespoon coconut oil

- 1 cup chopped broccoli florets

- 1 cup sliced red bell pepper

- 1/2 cup sliced sugar snap peas

- 1/2 cup sliced mushrooms

- 1 clove garlic, minced (optional, for those with mild FODMAP intolerance)

- 1/4 cup low-FODMAP soy sauce

- 1 tablespoon rice vinegar

- 1 tablespoon cornstarch

- 1/4 cup vegetable broth

- Cooked brown rice or quinoa (optional)

- Chopped fresh cilantro or basil (optional, for garnish)

INSTRUCTIONS

1. Heat coconut oil in a large skillet or wok over medium-high heat.

2. Add broccoli, red bell pepper, sugar snap peas, and mushrooms. Stir-fry for 5-7 minutes, or until vegetables are tender-crisp.

3. Add garlic (if using) and cook for 30 seconds more.

4. In a small bowl, whisk together soy sauce, rice vinegar, cornstarch, and vegetable broth. Stir until cornstarch is dissolved.

5. Pour the sauce into the skillet with the vegetables and bring to a simmer. Cook for 1-2 minutes, or until the sauce thickens slightly.

6. Serve stir-fry over cooked brown rice or quinoa (optional).

NOTES

- Adjust the amount of soy sauce to your taste and FODMAP tolerance.

- For a thicker sauce, add a bit more cornstarch slurry.

NUTRITIONAL INFORMATION (approximate per serving):

- Calories: 300 | Protein: 10g | Fat: 15g | Carbohydrates: 30g | Fiber: 5g | Sugar: 5g

Minestrone Soup

A hearty and comforting soup packed with vegetables. This low-FODMAP version is a classic Italian dish adapted for sensitive stomachs.

Prep Time: 20 minutes || **Cook Time:** 45 minutes || **Yield:** 4 servings

INGREDIENTS

- 1 tablespoon olive oil
- 1 leek, white part only, finely chopped
- 1 carrot, diced
- 1 zucchini, diced
- 1 can (400g) crushed tomatoes
- 1 can (400g) cannellini beans, rinsed and drained

- 4 cups vegetable broth
- 1/2 teaspoon dried oregano
- 1/4 teaspoon red pepper flakes (optional)
- Salt and pepper to taste
- Gluten-free pasta (low-FODMAP)
- Fresh basil, for garnish (optional)

INSTRUCTIONS

1. Heat olive oil in a large pot over medium heat. Add leek, carrot, and zucchini, cook until softened, about 5 minutes.

2. Stir in crushed tomatoes, cannellini beans, vegetable broth, oregano, and red pepper flakes. Bring to a boil, then reduce heat and simmer for 30 minutes, or until vegetables are tender.

3. Cook gluten-free pasta according to package directions.

4. Add cooked pasta to the soup and simmer for a few minutes to heat through.

5. Season with salt and pepper to taste. Serve hot, garnished with fresh basil (optional).

NOTES

- For a thicker soup, puree a portion of the soup and return it to the pot.

- Serve with a slice of crusty gluten-free bread (low-FODMAP) for dipping.

- This soup can be made ahead of time and reheated.

NUTRITIONAL INFORMATION (approximate per serving):

- Calories: 250 | Protein: 10g | Fat: 5g | Carbohydrates: 40g | Fiber: 7g | Sugar: 5g

Penne Alla Vodka

A creamy and flavorful pasta dish that's perfect for a comforting meal. This vegan version uses plant-based alternatives for a delicious and satisfying experience.

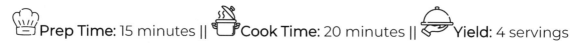 **Prep Time:** 15 minutes || **Cook Time:** 20 minutes || **Yield:** 4 servings

INGREDIENTS

- 8 ounces gluten-free penne pasta

- 1 tablespoon olive oil

- 1/4 cup vegan "vodka" (made from grapes or another low-FODMAP alcohol)

- 1/2 cup unsweetened almond milk

- 1/4 cup nutritional yeast

- 1 tablespoon tomato paste

- 1 teaspoon garlic powder (optional, for those with mild FODMAP intolerance)

- 1/4 teaspoon red pepper flakes (optional)

- Salt and pepper to taste

- Fresh basil, for garnish (optional)

INSTRUCTIONS

1. Cook pasta according to package directions. Reserve 1/2 cup pasta water.

2. While pasta cooks, heat olive oil in a large skillet over medium heat.

3. Add vegan vodka and cook for 30 seconds, until evaporated.

4. Stir in tomato paste and cook for 1 minute, until fragrant.

5. Add almond milk, nutritional yeast, garlic powder (if using), and red pepper flakes. Bring to a simmer.

6. Gradually add reserved pasta water, a little at a time, until desired sauce consistency is reached. Add cooked pasta to the sauce and toss to coat.

7. Serve immediately, garnished with fresh basil (optional).

NOTES

- For a thicker sauce, use more tomato paste or reduce the amount of almond milk.

- Serve with a side salad or garlic bread for a complete meal.

NUTRITIONAL INFORMATION (approximate per serving):

- Calories: 400 | Protein: 15g | Fat: 10g | Carbohydrates: 55g | Fiber: 3g | Sugar: 5g

Tuscan Bean Soup

A hearty and flavorful soup packed with protein and vegetables. This low-FODMAP version is a comforting and satisfying meal.

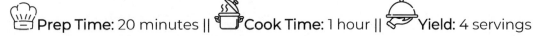

Prep Time: 20 minutes || **Cook Time:** 1 hour || **Yield:** 4 servings

INGREDIENTS

- 1 tablespoon olive oil

- 1 leek, white part only, finely chopped

- 1 carrot, finely diced

- 1 celery stalk, finely diced

- 1/2 teaspoon dried oregano

- 1/4 teaspoon red pepper flakes (optional)

- 1 can (15 oz) cannellini beans, rinsed and drained

- 1 can (15 oz) crushed tomatoes

- 4 cups vegetable broth

- 1 bay leaf

- Salt and pepper to taste

- Fresh basil, for garnish (optional)

- Gluten-free pasta (optional)

INSTRUCTIONS

1. Heat olive oil in a large pot over medium heat. Add leek, carrot, and celery, cook until softened, about 5 minutes.

2. Stir in oregano and red pepper flakes. Cook for 30 seconds more.

3. Add cannellini beans, crushed tomatoes, vegetable broth, and bay leaf to the pot. Bring to a boil, then reduce heat and simmer for at least 30 minutes, or up to 1 hour, for richer flavor.

4. Remove bay leaf. Season with salt and pepper to taste.

5. For a heartier soup, cook gluten-free pasta according to package directions and add to the soup. Serve hot, garnished with fresh basil (optional).

NOTES

- For a thicker soup, puree a portion of the soup and return it to the pot.

- Serve with a side of crusty bread (low-FODMAP) for dipping.

- This soup can be made ahead of time and reheated.

NUTRITIONAL INFORMATION (approximate per serving):

- Calories: 250 | Protein: 12g | Fat: 5g | Carbohydrates: 35g | Fiber: 7g | Sugar: 5g

Tortilla Salad Bowl

A fresh and vibrant meal packed with flavor and nutrients. This low-FODMAP version offers a satisfying and customizable dining experience.

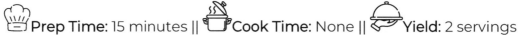 Prep Time: 15 minutes || Cook Time: None || Yield: 2 servings

INGREDIENTS

- 1 cup cooked black beans, rinsed and drained

- 1/2 cup corn (low-FODMAP, canned or frozen)

- 1/2 cup diced red bell pepper

- 1/4 cup diced red onion

- 1/4 cup chopped fresh cilantro

- 1/4 cup low-FODMAP tortilla chips, crushed

- Optional: avocado, sliced

For the dressing:

- 2 tablespoons lime juice

- 1 tablespoon olive oil

- 1/2 teaspoon ground cumin

- 1/4 teaspoon chili powder

- Salt and pepper to taste

INSTRUCTIONS

1. In a large bowl, combine black beans, corn, red bell pepper, red onion, and cilantro.

2. In a small bowl, whisk together lime juice, olive oil, cumin, chili powder, salt, and pepper to make the dressing.

3. Pour the dressing over the salad mixture and toss to coat evenly.

4. Divide the salad between two bowls and top with crushed tortilla chips and avocado slices, if desired.

NOTES

- Adjust the spice level by adding more or less chili powder.

- For a crunchier salad, add a handful of roasted sunflower seeds or pumpkin seeds.

- Serve with a side of guacamole (low-FODMAP) for extra flavor.

NUTRITIONAL INFORMATION (approximate per serving):

- Calories: 300 | Protein: 12g | Fat: 10g | Carbohydrates: 35g | Fiber: 8g | Sugar: 5g

Quinoa Veggie Bowl

A versatile and nutritious meal, this quinoa bowl can be customized with your favorite low-FODMAP vegetables.

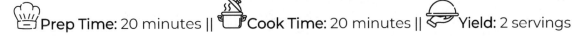

Prep Time: 20 minutes || **Cook Time:** 20 minutes || **Yield:** 2 servings

INGREDIENTS

- 1 cup quinoa, rinsed

- 2 cups vegetable broth

- 1/2 cup mixed bell peppers, diced

- 1/2 cup broccoli florets

- 1/4 cup sliced carrots

- 1/4 cup edamame, shelled

- 2 green onions, thinly sliced

- 2 tablespoons low-sodium soy sauce (tamari)

- 1 tablespoon sesame oil

- 1 teaspoon rice vinegar

- Salt and pepper to taste

INSTRUCTIONS

1. In a medium saucepan, combine quinoa and vegetable broth. Bring to a boil, then reduce heat, cover, and simmer for 15-20 minutes, or until quinoa is fluffy and liquid is absorbed.

2. While quinoa cooks, heat a large skillet over medium heat with a drizzle of sesame oil. Add bell peppers, broccoli, and carrots. Cook until tender-crisp.

3. Stir in edamame and cook for an additional minute.

4. In a small bowl, whisk together soy sauce and rice vinegar.

5. Combine cooked quinoa, sautéed vegetables, and edamame in a large bowl. Pour the soy sauce mixture over the top and toss to coat. Garnish with green onions and serve.

NOTES

- You can add other low-FODMAP vegetables to this bowl, such as zucchini, snow peas, or mushrooms.

- For a heartier meal, add a protein source like tofu or chickpeas.

- Serve with a side of avocado or a dollop of hummus for extra flavor and nutrients.

NUTRITIONAL INFORMATION (approximate per serving):

- Calories: 350 | Protein: 8g | Fat: 10g | Carbohydrates: 50g | Fiber: 5g | Sugar: 3g

Spaghetti Bolognese

A hearty and flavorful plant-based bolognese that's perfect for a comforting meal. This recipe is packed with vegetables and free from high-FODMAP ingredients.

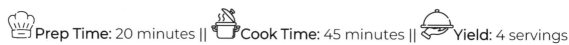 **Prep Time:** 20 minutes || **Cook Time:** 45 minutes || **Yield:** 4 servings

INGREDIENTS

- 1 tablespoon olive oil

- 1 large carrot, finely diced

- 1 leek, white part only, finely chopped

- 2 cloves garlic, minced (optional, for those with mild FODMAP intolerance)

- 1 teaspoon dried oregano

- 1/2 teaspoon dried basil

- Pinch of red pepper flakes (optional)

- 1 can (400g) crushed tomatoes

- 1 can (400g) lentils, rinsed and drained

- 1/4 cup vegetable broth

- 1 tablespoon tomato paste

- Salt and pepper to taste

- Gluten-free spaghetti

INSTRUCTIONS

1. Heat olive oil in a large skillet over medium heat. Add carrot and leek, cook until softened, about 5 minutes. Add garlic (if using), oregano, basil, and red pepper flakes, cook for 30 seconds more.

2. Stir in crushed tomatoes, lentils, vegetable broth, and tomato paste. Bring to a simmer, reduce heat, and let simmer for at least 30 minutes, or up to 1 hour, for richer flavor.

3. Cook gluten-free spaghetti. Serve the bolognese sauce over cooked spaghetti.

NOTES

- For a thicker sauce, reduce the cooking time or blend a portion of the sauce.

- Adjust the spices to your taste.

- Serve with grated vegan parmesan cheese (low-FODMAP certified) for extra flavor.

- This recipe can be prepared in advance and reheated.

NUTRITIONAL INFORMATION (approximate per serving):

- Calories: 400 | Protein: 15g | Fat: 10g | Carbohydrates: 55g | Fiber: 10g | Sugar: 5g

Green Bean Casserole

A classic comfort food with a low-FODMAP twist. This creamy and flavorful casserole is perfect for holidays or any special occasion.

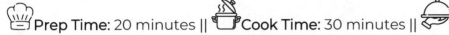 **Prep Time:** 20 minutes || **Cook Time:** 30 minutes || **Yield:** 4 servings

INGREDIENTS

- 1 pound fresh green beans, trimmed

- 1 can (10.5 oz) cream of mushroom soup (low-FODMAP or homemade)

- 1/2 cup unsweetened almond milk

- 1/4 cup gluten-free breadcrumbs

- 2 tablespoons vegan butter or olive oil

- 1/4 teaspoon garlic powder (optional)

- Salt and pepper to taste

INSTRUCTIONS

1. Preheat oven to 350°F (175°C).

2. Cook green beans in boiling salted water until tender-crisp, about 5 minutes. Drain and rinse with cold water.

3. In a large bowl, combine cooked green beans, cream of mushroom soup, almond milk, and garlic powder (if using). Stir until well combined.

4. Pour the mixture into a greased baking dish.

5. In a small skillet, melt vegan butter or olive oil over medium heat. Add breadcrumbs and cook until golden brown, stirring frequently.

6. Sprinkle breadcrumbs over the green bean mixture.

7. Bake for 20-25 minutes, or until bubbly and golden brown.

NOTES

- For a homemade cream of mushroom soup, sauté mushrooms in olive oil, then blend with vegetable broth, cornstarch, and almond milk until smooth.

- To make this dish gluten-free, use gluten-free breadcrumbs.

- For a richer flavor, add a pinch of nutmeg or thyme.

NUTRITIONAL INFORMATION (approximate per serving):

- Calories: 250 | Protein: 5g | Fat: 12g | Carbohydrates: 25g | Fiber: 4g | Sugar: 3g

Pumpkin Coconut Curry

A warming and comforting curry packed with flavor. This low-FODMAP version is rich in vegetables and perfect for a satisfying meal.

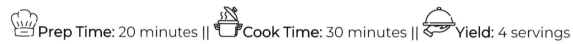 **Prep Time:** 20 minutes || **Cook Time:** 30 minutes || **Yield:** 4 servings

INGREDIENTS

- 1 tablespoon coconut oil

- 1 onion, finely chopped

- 1 inch piece of ginger, grated

- 2 cloves garlic, minced (optional, for those with mild FODMAP intolerance)

- 1 teaspoon ground coriander

- 1 teaspoon ground cumin

- 1/2 teaspoon turmeric

- 1/4 teaspoon red pepper flakes (optional)

- 1 can (400g) coconut milk

- 1 can (400g) chopped tomatoes

- 400g pumpkin, peeled and cubed

- 1/2 teaspoon salt

- 1/4 teaspoon black pepper

- Fresh cilantro, for garnish (optional)

- Cooked brown rice or cauliflower rice, to serve

INSTRUCTIONS

1. Heat coconut oil in a large pot or Dutch oven over medium heat. Add onion and cook until softened, about 5 minutes.

2. Stir in ginger, garlic (if using), coriander, cumin, turmeric, and red pepper flakes. Cook for 30 seconds more.

3. Add coconut milk, chopped tomatoes, and pumpkin to the pot. Bring to a boil, then reduce heat and simmer for 20-25 minutes, or until pumpkin is tender. Season with salt and pepper to taste.

5. Serve over cooked brown rice or cauliflower rice, garnished with fresh cilantro (optional).

NOTES

- For a thicker curry, use a combination of coconut milk and coconut cream.

- Serve with a side of naan bread (low-FODMAP) for a complete meal.

NUTRITIONAL INFORMATION (approximate per serving):

- Calories: 350 | Protein: 8g | Fat: 20g | Carbohydrates: 35g | Fiber: 5g | Sugar: 10g

Sesame Tofu with Sides

This dish offers a protein-packed main with versatile side options. The tofu is coated in a flavorful sesame sauce, and the sides can be customized based on your preference.

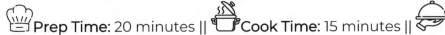 **Prep Time:** 20 minutes || **Cook Time:** 15 minutes || **Yield:** 2 servings

INGREDIENTS

For the Tofu:

- 1 block extra-firm tofu, pressed and cubed

- 2 tablespoons cornstarch

- 2 tablespoons soy sauce (low-sodium, tamari)

- 1 tablespoon sesame oil

- 1 teaspoon rice vinegar

- 1/2 teaspoon ginger powder

- Sesame seeds, for garnish

For the Sides:

- 1 cup cooked brown rice (low-FODMAP)

- 1/2 cucumber, julienned

- 1/4 cup shredded carrots

- Optional: steamed broccoli or stir-fried bok choy

INSTRUCTIONS

1. Press the tofu to remove excess water. Cut into cubes. Combine cornstarch, soy sauce, sesame oil, rice vinegar, and ginger powder in a bowl. Toss tofu cubes in this mixture to coat.

2. Heat a skillet with a drizzle of oil over medium heat. Cook tofu cubes until golden brown on all sides.

3. Serve the sesame tofu over a bed of brown rice. Top with cucumber, carrots, and your choice of side vegetables. Garnish with sesame seeds.

NOTES

- For additional flavor, you can marinate the tofu in the sauce for 15-30 minutes before cooking.

- To make this dish spicier, add a dash of red pepper flakes to the tofu marinade.

- Customize the side dishes based on your preferences and dietary needs.

NUTRITIONAL INFORMATION (approximate per serving):

- Calories: 400 | Protein: 20g | Fat: 15g | Carbohydrates: 40g | Fiber: 4g | Sugar: 3g

Veggie Burger II

A hearty and flavorful plant-based burger with a different twist. This version uses lentils for a protein-packed and satisfying meal.

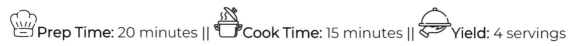 **Prep Time:** 20 minutes || **Cook Time:** 15 minutes || **Yield:** 4 servings

INGREDIENTS

- 1 can (15 oz) green lentils, rinsed and drained

- 1/2 cup cooked brown rice or quinoa

- 1/2 cup grated zucchini

- 1/4 cup chopped celery

- 1/4 cup breadcrumbs (gluten-free and low-FODMAP)

- 1 tablespoon ground flaxseed mixed with 3 tablespoons water (flax egg)

- 1 teaspoon smoked paprika

- 1/2 teaspoon ground coriander

- 1/4 teaspoon chili powder

- Salt and pepper to taste

INSTRUCTIONS

1. In a large bowl, mash lentils with a fork, leaving some whole lentils for texture.

2. Add cooked rice or quinoa, grated zucchini, chopped celery, breadcrumbs, flax egg, smoked paprika, coriander, chili powder, salt, and pepper to the lentils. Mix well until combined.

3. Shape the mixture into four patties.

4. Heat a large skillet over medium heat with a drizzle of olive oil.

5. Cook patties for 5-7 minutes per side, or until golden brown and cooked through.

6. Serve on a low-FODMAP bun with your favorite toppings, such as lettuce, tomato, and vegan mayo.

NOTES

- To make the patties hold together better, refrigerate the mixture for 30 minutes before shaping.

- Serve with a side of sweet potato fries or a green salad for a complete meal.

NUTRITIONAL INFORMATION (approximate per serving):

- Calories: 250 | Protein: 15g | Fat: 5g | Carbohydrates: 30g | Fiber: 6g | Sugar: 3g

Adobo Tempeh Meatballs

These savory and flavorful tempeh meatballs capture the essence of Filipino adobo without compromising on digestive comfort. Packed with protein and low in FODMAPs, they're a satisfying and healthy meal option.

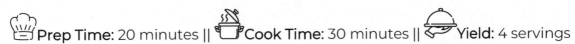

Prep Time: 20 minutes || **Cook Time:** 30 minutes || **Yield:** 4 servings

INGREDIENTS

- 1 block tempeh, crumbled

- 1/2 cup breadcrumbs (gluten-free and low-FODMAP)

- 1/4 cup unsweetened almond milk

- 1 tablespoon low-FODMAP soy sauce

- 1 teaspoon garlic powder

- 1/2 teaspoon ground cumin

- 1/4 teaspoon black pepper

- 1 tablespoon olive oil

For the adobo sauce:

- 1 tablespoon low-FODMAP soy sauce

- 1 tablespoon apple cider vinegar

- 1 teaspoon brown sugar

- 1/2 teaspoon ground black pepper

INSTRUCTIONS

1. Preheat oven to 375°F (190°C). Line a baking sheet with parchment paper.

2. In a large bowl, combine crumbled tempeh, breadcrumbs, almond milk, soy sauce, garlic powder, cumin, and black pepper. Mix well until combined.

3. Shape the mixture into small meatballs, about 1 inch in diameter.

4. In a small bowl, whisk together the adobo sauce ingredients.

5. Arrange meatballs on the prepared baking sheet and brush with the adobo sauce.

6. Bake for 25-30 minutes, or until golden brown and cooked through.

7. Serve hot with your favorite low-FODMAP side dishes, such as cauliflower rice or zucchini noodles.

NOTES

- For a richer flavor, marinate the tempeh mixture for 30 minutes before shaping into meatballs.

- Adjust the amount of soy sauce according to your taste and FODMAP tolerance.

- Serve with a side of steamed green beans or roasted sweet potatoes for a complete meal.

NUTRITIONAL INFORMATION (approximate per serving):

- Calories: 250 | Protein: 20g | Fat: 10g | Carbohydrates: 25g | Fiber: 5g | Sugar: 5g

Baked Zucchini and Squash

A simple yet flavorful side dish that's perfect for any meal. This low-FODMAP recipe highlights the natural sweetness of zucchini and squash.

Prep Time: 15 minutes || **Cook Time:** 30-35 minutes || **Yield:** 4 servings

INGREDIENTS

- 1 medium zucchini, sliced

- 1 medium yellow squash, sliced

- 2 tablespoons olive oil

- 1 teaspoon dried oregano

- 1/2 teaspoon garlic powder (optional, for those with mild FODMAP intolerance)

- Salt and pepper to taste

INSTRUCTIONS

1. Preheat oven to 400°F (200°C). Line a baking sheet with parchment paper.

2. In a large bowl, combine zucchini, yellow squash, olive oil, oregano, garlic powder (if using), salt, and pepper. Toss to coat.

3. Spread the vegetable mixture in a single layer on the prepared baking sheet.

4. Bake for 30-35 minutes, or until vegetables are tender and slightly browned.

5. Serve hot as a side dish or as a base for other dishes.

NOTES

- For added flavor, sprinkle with nutritional yeast or lemon zest before serving.

- You can use other summer squash varieties, such as pattypan or crookneck.

- Serve with hummus or tahini for a more substantial side dish.

NUTRITIONAL INFORMATION (approximate per serving):

- Calories: 100 | Protein: 2g | Fat: 7g | Carbohydrates: 8g | Fiber: 2g | Sugar: 3g

Cold Sesame Noodle Salad

A refreshing and light dish perfect for warmer weather. This noodle salad is packed with flavor and nutrients.

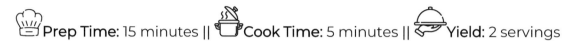 **Prep Time:** 15 minutes || **Cook Time:** 5 minutes || **Yield:** 2 servings

INGREDIENTS

- 8 oz rice noodles (gluten-free, low-FODMAP)

- 1/2 cucumber, julienned

- 1/4 cup shredded carrots

- 1/4 cup sliced red bell pepper

- 2 green onions, thinly sliced

- 1/4 cup roasted sesame seeds

For the dressing:

- 2 tablespoons tahini

- 1 tablespoon rice vinegar

- 1 tablespoon soy sauce (low-sodium, tamari)

- 1 teaspoon sesame oil

- 1/2 teaspoon grated ginger

- 1/4 teaspoon red pepper flakes (optional)

INSTRUCTIONS

1. Cook rice noodles according to package directions. Rinse under cold water to stop the cooking process. Drain well.

2. In a large bowl, combine cooked noodles, cucumber, carrots, red bell pepper, and green onions.

3. In a small bowl, whisk together tahini, rice vinegar, soy sauce, sesame oil, ginger, and red pepper flakes until smooth.

4. Pour the dressing over the noodle mixture and toss to coat evenly.

5. Sprinkle with sesame seeds and serve immediately.

NOTES

- For added protein, consider adding tofu or edamame.

- Serve chilled for a refreshing summer meal.

NUTRITIONAL INFORMATION (approximate per serving):

- Calories: 300 | Protein: 8g | Fat: 12g | Carbohydrates: 40g | Fiber: 2g | Sugar: 3g

Veggie & Avocado Roll Ups

These fresh and flavorful roll-ups are perfect for a quick and healthy lunch or snack. Packed with vegetables and protein, they are a satisfying and low-FODMAP option.

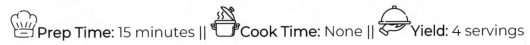 **Prep Time:** 15 minutes || **Cook Time:** None || **Yield:** 4 servings

INGREDIENTS

- 4 large lettuce leaves (e.g., romaine or iceberg)

- 1/2 avocado, mashed

- 1/4 cup hummus (low-FODMAP)

- 1/4 cup shredded carrots

- 1/4 cup cucumber, sliced

- 1/4 cup red bell pepper, diced

- Optional: a sprinkle of toasted sesame seeds

INSTRUCTIONS

1. Lay out the lettuce leaves on a flat surface.

2. Spread a layer of hummus on each lettuce leaf.

3. Top with mashed avocado, carrots, cucumber, and red bell pepper.

4. Roll up the lettuce leaves tightly to form wraps.

5. Sprinkle with sesame seeds, if desired.

NOTES

- You can customize these roll-ups with your favorite low-FODMAP vegetables.

- For extra protein, add grilled tofu or chickpeas.

- Serve with a side of hummus or your favorite low-FODMAP dip.

NUTRITIONAL INFORMATION (approximate per serving):

- Calories: 150 | Protein: 3g | Fat: 10g | Carbohydrates: 10g | Fiber: 3g | Sugar: 2g

Spinach and Mandarin Orange Salad

A refreshing and light salad packed with nutrients. This low-FODMAP option is perfect as a side dish or a light meal.

Prep Time: 10 minutes || **Cook Time:** None || **Yield:** 2 servings

INGREDIENTS

- 4 cups fresh spinach, washed and dried

- 1/2 cup mandarin oranges, segmented

- 1/4 cup sliced almonds (optional)

- 1/4 cup dried cranberries (check for low-FODMAP certification)

For the dressing:

- 2 tablespoons olive oil

- 1 tablespoon balsamic vinegar

- 1 teaspoon Dijon mustard

- 1/2 teaspoon honey (optional)

- Salt and pepper to taste

INSTRUCTIONS

1. In a large bowl, combine spinach, mandarin oranges, almonds, and cranberries.

2. In a small bowl, whisk together olive oil, balsamic vinegar, Dijon mustard, honey (if using), salt, and pepper until emulsified.

3. Pour dressing over the salad and toss to coat evenly.

4. Serve immediately.

NOTES

- For a crunchier salad, add a handful of toasted sunflower seeds.

- Adjust the sweetness of the dressing by adding more or less honey.

- This salad can be prepared ahead of time, but the dressing should be added just before serving to keep the spinach fresh.

NUTRITIONAL INFORMATION (approximate per serving):

- Calories: 200 | Protein: 4g | Fat: 12g | Carbohydrates: 15g | Fiber: 2g | Sugar: 8g

Spinach and Quinoa Stuffed Peppers

A hearty and healthy meal packed with nutrients. These stuffed peppers are a satisfying and flavorful option.

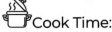**Prep Time:** 25 minutes || 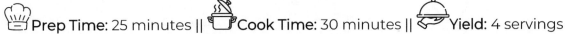**Cook Time:** 30 minutes || 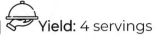**Yield:** 4 servings

INGREDIENTS

- 4 large bell peppers

- 1 cup cooked quinoa (low-FODMAP)

- 2 cups fresh spinach, chopped

- 1/2 cup diced red onion

- 1/4 cup sun-dried tomatoes (packed in oil, drained and chopped)

- 1/4 cup vegan parmesan cheese (low-FODMAP)

- 2 cloves garlic, minced (optional, for those with mild FODMAP intolerance)

- 1 tablespoon olive oil

- Salt and pepper to taste

INSTRUCTIONS

1. Preheat oven to 375°F (190°C).

2. Cut the tops off the bell peppers and remove the seeds.

3. In a large skillet, heat olive oil over medium heat. Add onion and garlic (if using), and cook until softened.

4. Add spinach and cook until wilted. Remove from heat and let cool slightly.

5. Combine cooked quinoa, spinach, sun-dried tomatoes, vegan parmesan cheese, salt, and pepper in a large bowl.

6. Stuff the bell pepper halves with the quinoa mixture.

7. Place stuffed peppers in a baking dish and bake for 30 minutes, or until peppers are tender.

NOTES

- For a richer flavor, add a spoonful of tahini or nutritional yeast to the filling.

- Serve with a side salad or a dollop of vegan yogurt for a complete meal.

NUTRITIONAL INFORMATION (approximate per serving):

- Calories: 250 | Protein: 10g | Fat: 8g | Carbohydrates: 35g | Fiber: 5g | Sugar: 5g

Golden Polenta Fries with Sage and Thyme

These crispy and flavorful polenta fries are a perfect low-FODMAP alternative to traditional potato fries. The addition of sage and thyme gives them a delightful herby twist.

Prep Time: 20 minutes + cooling time || **Cook Time:** 20-25 minutes || **Yield:** 4 servings

INGREDIENTS

- 2 cups vegetable broth

- 1 cup polenta

- 1 teaspoon dried sage

- 1 teaspoon dried thyme

- 1/2 teaspoon garlic powder (optional)

- Salt and pepper to taste

- Olive oil, for frying

INSTRUCTIONS

1. Bring vegetable broth to a boil in a medium saucepan. Gradually whisk in polenta until smooth. Reduce heat to low and simmer for 15-20 minutes, or until polenta is thick and creamy, stirring occasionally.

2. Stir in sage, thyme, garlic powder, salt, and pepper.

3. Pour the polenta mixture into a greased baking dish. Cover with plastic wrap and refrigerate for at least 30 minutes or overnight to firm up.

4. Cut the polenta into fry-shaped sticks.

5. Heat olive oil in a large skillet over medium heat.

6. Fry the polenta fries in batches until golden brown and crispy on all sides.

7. Drain on paper towels and season with additional salt and pepper, if desired.

NOTES

- For a healthier option, bake the polenta fries instead of frying them. Preheat oven to 400°F (200°C) and bake for 20-25 minutes, or until golden brown and crispy.

- Serve with your favorite low-FODMAP dipping sauce, such as marinara sauce or hummus.

NUTRITIONAL INFORMATION (approximate per serving):

- Calories: 250 | Protein: 5g | Fat: 10g | Carbohydrates: 35g | Fiber: 2g | Sugar: 1g

SNACKS, DESSERTS & SIDES

Vanilla Custard

A creamy and comforting dessert that's perfect for satisfying your sweet tooth. This vegan custard is rich in flavor and free from high-FODMAP ingredients.

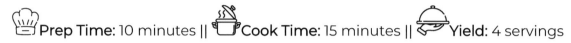 **Prep Time:** 10 minutes || **Cook Time:** 15 minutes || **Yield:** 4 servings

INGREDIENTS

- 2 cups unsweetened almond milk

- 1/4 cup cornstarch

- 1/4 cup maple syrup

- 1 teaspoon vanilla extract

- Pinch of salt

INSTRUCTIONS

1. In a medium saucepan, whisk together almond milk, cornstarch, maple syrup, vanilla extract, and salt.

2. Cook over medium heat, stirring constantly, until the mixture thickens and comes to a boil.

3. Reduce heat and simmer for 1 minute, stirring continuously.

4. Remove from heat and pour into individual serving dishes.

5. Let cool completely before serving.

NOTES

- For a richer custard, use full-fat coconut milk instead of almond milk.

- You can add a pinch of xanthan gum for a smoother texture.

- Serve with fresh berries or a sprinkle of cinnamon for added flavor.

- Store leftovers in the refrigerator for up to 3 days.

NUTRITIONAL INFORMATION (approximate per serving):

- Calories: 150 | Protein: 2g | Fat: 5g | Carbohydrates: 25g | Fiber: 1g | Sugar: 10g

Marinara Sauce

A classic Italian sauce, adapted for those following a low-FODMAP diet. This marinara is packed with flavor and perfect for pasta or as a pizza base.

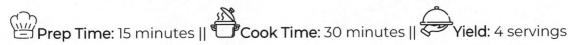

Prep Time: 15 minutes || **Cook Time:** 30 minutes || **Yield:** 4 servings

INGREDIENTS

- 1 tablespoon olive oil

- 1 onion, finely chopped

- 2 cloves garlic, minced (optional, for those with mild FODMAP intolerance)

- 1 can (28 ounces) crushed tomatoes

- 1 teaspoon dried oregano

- 1/2 teaspoon dried basil

- 1/4 teaspoon red pepper flakes (optional)

- Salt and pepper to taste

INSTRUCTIONS

1. Heat olive oil in a large saucepan over medium heat. Add onion and garlic (if using) and cook until softened, about 5 minutes.

2. Stir in crushed tomatoes, oregano, basil, and red pepper flakes. Bring to a simmer.

3. Reduce heat and let simmer for at least 30 minutes, or up to an hour, for a richer flavor.

4. Season with salt and pepper to taste.

NOTES

- For a thicker sauce, simmer for a longer period or use a tomato paste base.

- Adjust the spice level by adding more or less red pepper flakes.

- Serve over your favorite gluten-free pasta or use as a pizza sauce base.

- This sauce can be made ahead of time and stored in the refrigerator for up to a week.

NUTRITIONAL INFORMATION (approximate per serving):

- Calories: 100 | Protein: 2g | Fat: 5g | Carbohydrates: 10g | Fiber: 2g | Sugar: 5g

Green Smoothie

A refreshing and nutrient-packed smoothie to kickstart your day. This green delight is packed with vitamins and minerals, and is gentle on the digestive system.

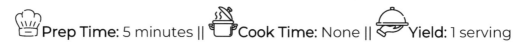 **Prep Time:** 5 minutes || **Cook Time:** None || **Yield:** 1 serving

INGREDIENTS

- 1 cup spinach or kale

- 1/2 ripe banana (or a low-FODMAP fruit like pineapple or berries)

- 1/2 cup unsweetened almond milk (or other low-FODMAP milk)

- 1 tablespoon chia seeds

- 1/4 avocado (optional, for creaminess)

- 1 tablespoon lemon juice

- A handful of ice cubes

INSTRUCTIONS

1. Combine all ingredients in a blender.

2. Blend until smooth and creamy.

3. Adjust sweetness to taste by adding more banana or a drizzle of maple syrup.

NOTES

- For a sweeter smoothie, use a low-FODMAP fruit like pineapple or berries instead of banana.

- Experiment with different greens like romaine lettuce or collard greens.

- Add a scoop of protein powder for an extra boost (ensure it's low-FODMAP).

- For a thicker smoothie, use frozen banana or add more ice cubes.

NUTRITIONAL INFORMATION (approximate per serving):

- Calories: 200 | Protein: 5g | Fat: 8g | Carbohydrates: 25g | Fiber: 5g | Sugar: 10g

Blueberry Muffins

These fluffy and flavorful muffins are a delicious treat that's gentle on the digestive system. Packed with antioxidants from blueberries, they're a perfect start to your day.

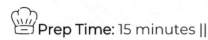**Prep Time:** 15 minutes || 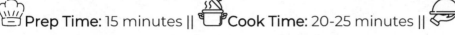**Cook Time:** 20-25 minutes || 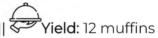**Yield:** 12 muffins

INGREDIENTS

- 1 cup gluten-free oat flour

- 1/2 teaspoon baking powder

- 1/4 teaspoon baking soda

- Pinch of salt

- 1/4 cup maple syrup

- 1/2 cup unsweetened almond milk

- 1 tablespoon apple cider vinegar

- 1 tablespoon flaxseed meal mixed with 3 tablespoons water (flax egg)

- 1 teaspoon vanilla extract

- 1 cup fresh blueberries

- Optional topping: additional blueberries

INSTRUCTIONS

1. Preheat oven to 350°F (175°C). Line a muffin tin with paper liners.

2. In a large bowl, whisk together oat flour, baking powder, baking soda, and salt.

3. In a separate bowl, whisk together maple syrup, almond milk, apple cider vinegar, flax egg, and vanilla extract.

4. Combine wet ingredients with dry ingredients until just combined. Gently fold in blueberries. Divide batter evenly among muffin cups.

5. Bake for 20-25 minutes, or until a toothpick inserted into the center comes out clean.

6. Let cool in the muffin tin for a few minutes before transferring to a wire rack to cool completely.

NOTES

- For a richer flavor, use coconut oil instead of flax egg.

- To avoid muffins sticking to the pan, lightly grease the muffin tin before lining with paper liners.

NUTRITIONAL INFORMATION (approximate per serving):

- Calories: 150 | Protein: 3g | Fat: 5g | Carbohydrates: 25g | Fiber: 2g | Sugar: 10g

Fruit Crumble Bars

A delightful treat that's both satisfying and gentle on the digestive system. These crumble bars offer a delicious balance of sweet and crumbly textures.

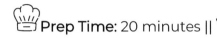**Prep Time:** 20 minutes || 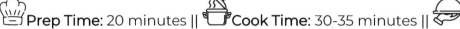**Cook Time:** 30-35 minutes || 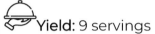**Yield:** 9 servings

INGREDIENTS

For the crumble topping:

- 1 cup gluten-free oat flour

- 1/2 cup almond flour

- 1/4 cup coconut sugar

- 1/4 teaspoon cinnamon

- Pinch of salt

- 1/4 cup coconut oil, melted

For the fruit filling:

- 2 cups mixed berries (strawberries, raspberries, blueberries - use low-FODMAP serving sizes)

- 1/4 cup maple syrup

- 1 tablespoon cornstarch

- Juice of 1/2 lemon

INSTRUCTIONS

1. Preheat oven to 350°F (175°C). Grease a 9x9 inch baking dish.

2. In a medium bowl, combine oat flour, almond flour, coconut sugar, cinnamon, and salt. Stir in melted coconut oil until crumbly.

3. In a large bowl, combine berries, maple syrup, cornstarch, and lemon juice. Toss to coat.

4. Spread the fruit filling evenly in the prepared baking dish. Sprinkle the crumble topping over the fruit.

5. Bake for 30-35 minutes, or until the crumble is golden brown and the fruit is bubbling.

6. Let cool completely before cutting into bars.

NOTES

- For a gluten-free and nut-free option, use a gluten-free oat flour that is also certified nut-free.

- For a thicker filling, use a combination of cornstarch and arrowroot flour.

NUTRITIONAL INFORMATION (approximate per serving):

- Calories: 250 | Protein: 4g | Fat: 12g | Carbohydrates: 30g | Fiber: 4g | Sugar: 15g

Vodka Pasta Sauce

This creamy and flavorful sauce captures the essence of a classic vodka pasta without the high-FODMAP ingredients. It's a perfect base for your favorite gluten-free pasta.

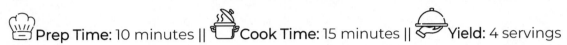 **Prep Time:** 10 minutes || **Cook Time:** 15 minutes || **Yield:** 4 servings

INGREDIENTS

- 1/4 cup tomato paste

- 1/4 cup unsweetened almond milk

- 1 tablespoon gluten-free vodka

- 1 teaspoon garlic-infused olive oil (low-FODMAP)

- 1/4 teaspoon red pepper flakes (optional)

- Salt and pepper to taste

- Fresh basil, for garnish (optional)

INSTRUCTIONS

1. In a medium saucepan, heat tomato paste and garlic-infused olive oil over medium heat for about 1 minute, stirring constantly.

2. Gradually whisk in almond milk until the sauce is smooth.

3. Add vodka and red pepper flakes. Let simmer for 2-3 minutes to allow the alcohol to evaporate.

4. Season with salt and pepper to taste.

5. Serve over your favorite gluten-free pasta. Garnish with fresh basil, if desired.

NOTES

- For a thicker sauce, use a combination of almond milk and cornstarch.

- Adjust the spice level by adding more or less red pepper flakes.

- Serve with additional toppings such as grated vegan parmesan (low-FODMAP) or chopped sun-dried tomatoes.

NUTRITIONAL INFORMATION (approximate per serving):

- Calories: 150 | Protein: 2g | Fat: 5g | Carbohydrates: 15g | Fiber: 1g | Sugar: 5g

Magnum Ice Cream

A refreshing and indulgent treat that's perfect for a hot day. This homemade version of a classic ice cream bar is packed with flavor and free from high-FODMAP ingredients.

To create the classic Magnum shape, you'll need ice pop molds.

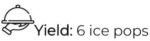 **Prep Time:** 20 minutes, plus freezing time || **Yield:** 6 ice pops

INGREDIENTS

For the ice cream:

- 1 can (400ml) full-fat coconut milk, chilled

- 1/4 cup maple syrup

- 1 teaspoon vanilla extract

For the chocolate coating:

- 100g dark chocolate (low-FODMAP), chopped

- 1 tablespoon coconut oil

INSTRUCTIONS

1. Line an ice pop mold with sticks.

2. In a chilled bowl, whisk the coconut cream until it becomes thick and fluffy.

3. Gradually whisk in maple syrup and vanilla extract until combined.

4. Divide the ice cream mixture evenly among the ice pop molds.

5. Freeze for at least 6 hours, or overnight.

6. Melt dark chocolate and coconut oil together in a double boiler or microwave in short bursts, stirring until smooth.

7. Remove ice pops from the mold and dip the frozen ice cream into the melted chocolate, allowing excess to drip off.

8. Insert the ice pop sticks back into the chocolate-coated ice cream.

9. Place the coated ice pops back in the freezer to set the chocolate.

NOTES

- For a richer flavor, use dark chocolate with a higher cocoa content.

- You can experiment with different flavors by adding extracts or purees to the ice cream base.

- For a smoother texture, strain the coconut cream before using.

- Store homemade Magnum ice creams in the freezer for up to 2 weeks.

NUTRITIONAL INFORMATION (approximate per serving):

- Calories: 250 | Protein: 2g | Fat: 18g | Carbohydrates: 15g | Fiber: 1g | Sugar: 10g

Strawberry Crumble

A classic dessert with a low-FODMAP twist. This fruity crumble is perfect for satisfying your sweet tooth without digestive discomfort.

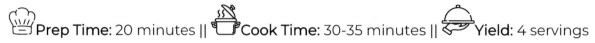 **Prep Time:** 20 minutes || **Cook Time:** 30-35 minutes || **Yield:** 4 servings

INGREDIENTS

For the strawberry filling:

- 2 cups fresh strawberries, hulled and sliced

- 1 tablespoon cornstarch

- 1/4 cup maple syrup

- 1 teaspoon lemon juice

For the crumble topping:

- 1/2 cup gluten-free oat flour

- 1/4 cup almond flour

- 1/4 cup coconut sugar

- 1/4 teaspoon cinnamon

- Pinch of salt

- 1/4 cup coconut oil, melted

INSTRUCTIONS

1. Preheat oven to 350°F (175°C). Grease a baking dish.

2. In a medium bowl, combine strawberries, cornstarch, maple syrup, and lemon juice. Toss to coat.

3. In a separate bowl, combine oat flour, almond flour, coconut sugar, cinnamon, and salt. Stir in melted coconut oil until crumbly. Pour the strawberry filling into the prepared baking dish.

4. Sprinkle the crumble topping evenly over the strawberries.

5. Bake for 30-35 minutes, or until the crumble is golden brown and the strawberries are bubbling. Let cool slightly before serving.

NOTES

- For a thicker filling, use a combination of cornstarch and arrowroot flour.

- Serve warm with a scoop of low-FODMAP ice cream for a decadent dessert.

NUTRITIONAL INFORMATION (approximate per serving):

- Calories: 250 | Protein: 3g | Fat: 12g | Carbohydrates: 30g | Fiber: 3g | Sugar: 15g

Key Lime Cheesecake

A refreshing and tangy dessert that's perfect for any occasion. This vegan version uses plant-based ingredients and is completely free of high-FODMAPs. This recipe requires a low-FODMAP cookie crust or a store-bought option.

Prep Time: 30 minutes, plus chilling time || 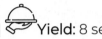**Yield:** 8 servings

INGREDIENTS

For the crust:

- 1 cup low-FODMAP cookie crumbs (e.g., gluten-free gingersnaps)

- 1/4 cup melted coconut oil

For the filling:

- 1 can (13.5 oz) full-fat coconut milk, chilled

- 1/2 cup lime juice (about 4 limes)

- 1/4 cup maple syrup

- 1 tablespoon cornstarch

- 1/4 teaspoon xanthan gum

- Zest of 1 lime

INSTRUCTIONS

1. Combine cookie crumbs and melted coconut oil in a bowl. Press the mixture into the bottom of a springform pan. Place in the refrigerator while preparing the filling.

2. In a chilled bowl, whisk the thickened coconut cream (from the top of the chilled coconut milk can) until stiff peaks form.

3. In a separate bowl, whisk together lime juice, maple syrup, cornstarch, xanthan gum, and lime zest.

4. Gently fold the lime mixture into the whipped coconut cream until combined.

5. Pour the filling over the prepared crust. Refrigerate for at least 4 hours, or overnight, to set.

NOTES

- For a thicker filling, use more cornstarch or xanthan gum.

- Adjust the sweetness to taste by adding more or less maple syrup.

- Decorate with fresh lime zest or a dollop of coconut whipped cream before serving.

NUTRITIONAL INFORMATION (approximate per serving):

- Calories: 250 | Protein: 2g | Fat: 18g | Carbohydrates: 20g | Fiber: 2g | Sugar: 12g

Sweet Potato Muffins

These muffins are a delicious and nutritious breakfast or snack option. The sweetness of the sweet potato combined with the spices create a delightful flavor.

Prep Time: 20 minutes || **Cook Time:** 20-25 minutes || **Yield:** 12 muffins

INGREDIENTS

- 1 large sweet potato, peeled and mashed
- 1 cup gluten-free oat flour
- 1/2 teaspoon baking powder
- 1/4 teaspoon baking soda
- 1/2 teaspoon cinnamon
- Pinch of nutmeg
- Pinch of salt
- 1/4 cup maple syrup
- 1/4 cup unsweetened almond milk
- Optional: raisins or cranberries (low-FODMAP)

INSTRUCTIONS

1. Preheat oven to 350°F (175°C). Line a muffin tin with paper liners.

2. In a large bowl, combine mashed sweet potato, oat flour, baking powder, baking soda, cinnamon, nutmeg, and salt.

3. Stir in maple syrup and almond milk until just combined. Fold in raisins or cranberries, if using.

4. Divide the batter evenly among the muffin liners.

5. Bake for 20-25 minutes, or until a toothpick inserted into the center comes out clean.

6. Let cool in the muffin tin for a few minutes before transferring to a wire rack to cool completely.

NOTES

- For a richer flavor, add a tablespoon of coconut oil or apple cider vinegar to the batter.

- You can top the muffins with a sprinkle of cinnamon sugar for added sweetness.

NUTRITIONAL INFORMATION (approximate per serving):

- Calories: 150 | Protein: 3g | Fat: 5g | Carbohydrates: 25g | Fiber: 2g | Sugar: 8g

Chocolate Pretzel Bars

A decadent treat that's perfect for satisfying your sweet and salty cravings. These bars are packed with flavor and are completely free of high-FODMAP ingredients. This recipe requires gluten-free pretzels that are low in FODMAPs.

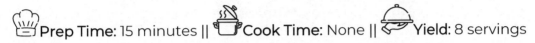 **Prep Time:** 15 minutes || **Cook Time:** None || **Yield:** 8 servings

INGREDIENTS

- 1 cup gluten-free pretzels, crushed

- 1/2 cup almond butter

- 1/4 cup maple syrup

- 1/4 cup cocoa powder

- Pinch of salt

INSTRUCTIONS

1. Line an 8x8 inch baking dish with parchment paper.

2. In a food processor, pulse the gluten-free pretzels until finely crushed.

3. In a separate bowl, combine almond butter, maple syrup, cocoa powder, and salt. Mix until smooth.

4. Add the crushed pretzels to the chocolate mixture and stir until combined.

5. Press the mixture evenly into the prepared baking dish.

6. Refrigerate for at least 1 hour to set.

7. Cut into bars and enjoy.

NOTES

- For a richer flavor, use dark chocolate cocoa powder.

- You can add chopped nuts (low-FODMAP) or dried fruit for extra texture.

- Store leftovers in the refrigerator for up to a week.

NUTRITIONAL INFORMATION (approximate per serving):

- Calories: 200 | Protein: 4g | Fat: 12g | Carbohydrates: 18g | Fiber: 2g | Sugar: 8g

Almond Butter Granola

This crunchy and flavorful granola is perfect for a satisfying breakfast or a healthy snack. Packed with nutrients and low in FODMAPs, it's a delicious way to start your day.

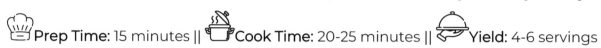 **Prep Time:** 15 minutes || **Cook Time:** 20-25 minutes || **Yield:** 4-6 servings

INGREDIENTS

- 2 cups gluten-free rolled oats
- 1/2 cup unsweetened coconut flakes
- 1/4 cup sliced almonds
- 1/4 cup pumpkin seeds
- 1/4 teaspoon cinnamon

- Pinch of salt
- 1/4 cup almond butter
- 1/4 cup maple syrup
- 1 tablespoon coconut oil, melted

INSTRUCTIONS

1. Preheat oven to 350°F (175°C). Line a baking sheet with parchment paper.

2. In a large bowl, combine oats, coconut flakes, almonds, pumpkin seeds, cinnamon, and salt.

3. In a separate bowl, whisk together almond butter, maple syrup, and melted coconut oil until smooth.

4. Pour the wet ingredients over the dry ingredients and stir until evenly coated.

5. Spread the granola mixture evenly on the prepared baking sheet.

6. Bake for 20-25 minutes, or until golden brown and crispy. Stir halfway through baking.

7. Let cool completely before storing in an airtight container.

NOTES

- For a nut-free option, omit the almonds and replace with sunflower seeds.
- Adjust sweetness to taste by adding more or less maple syrup.
- Store granola in an airtight container for up to 2 weeks.

NUTRITIONAL INFORMATION (approximate per serving):

- Calories: 250 | Protein: 6g | Fat: 12g | Carbohydrates: 30g | Fiber: 4g | Sugar: 8g

Dark Chocolate Granola

A decadent and satisfying breakfast or snack. This low-FODMAP granola is packed with rich chocolate flavor and crunchy texture.

Prep Time: 15 minutes || 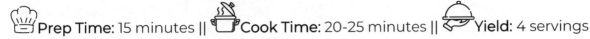**Cook Time:** 20-25 minutes || 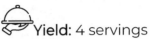**Yield:** 4 servings

INGREDIENTS

- 2 cups gluten-free rolled oats

- 1/2 cup unsweetened coconut flakes

- 1/4 cup sunflower seeds

- 1/4 cup pumpkin seeds

- 1/4 cup cocoa powder

- 1/4 cup maple syrup

- 1/4 cup coconut oil, melted

- 1/4 teaspoon salt

- 1/4 cup dark chocolate chips (low-FODMAP)

INSTRUCTIONS

1. Preheat oven to 350°F (175°C). Line a baking sheet with parchment paper.

2. In a large bowl, combine oats, coconut flakes, sunflower seeds, pumpkin seeds, and cocoa powder.

3. In a separate bowl, whisk together maple syrup, coconut oil, and salt.

4. Pour the wet ingredients over the dry ingredients and stir until evenly coated.

5. Spread the granola mixture evenly on the prepared baking sheet.

6. Bake for 20-25 minutes, or until golden brown and crispy. Stir halfway through baking.

7. Let cool completely, then stir in dark chocolate chips.

8. Store in an airtight container at room temperature.

NOTES

- For a nut-free option, omit the sunflower and pumpkin seeds.

- Adjust sweetness to taste by adding more or less maple syrup.

- Serve with low-FODMAP yogurt or plant-based milk for a complete breakfast.

NUTRITIONAL INFORMATION (approximate per serving):

- Calories: 250 | Protein: 5g | Fat: 12g | Carbohydrates: 30g | Fiber: 4g | Sugar: 8g

Lemon & Pineapple Tart

This recipe requires a low-FODMAP tart base, which can be store-bought or homemade.

Prep Time: 30 minutes || **Cook Time:** None || **Yield:** 8 servings

INGREDIENTS

For the filling:

- 1 cup fresh pineapple, diced

- 1/2 cup lemon juice

- 1/4 cup maple syrup

- 1 tablespoon cornstarch

- Pinch of salt

INSTRUCTIONS

1. Preheat oven to 350°F (175°C).

2. In a medium saucepan, combine pineapple, lemon juice, maple syrup, cornstarch, and salt.

3. Bring the mixture to a boil, stirring constantly. Reduce heat and simmer until thickened, about 5-7 minutes.

4. Remove from heat and let cool completely.

5. Pour the filling into a prepared low-FODMAP tart base.

6. Refrigerate for at least 2 hours to set.

NOTES

- For a thicker filling, use a combination of cornstarch and arrowroot flour.

- Adjust sweetness to taste by adding more or less maple syrup.

- Decorate with fresh pineapple chunks or lemon zest for a festive touch.

- Store leftovers in the refrigerator for up to 3 days.

NUTRITIONAL INFORMATION (approximate per serving):

- Calories: 150 | Protein: 1g | Fat: 5g | Carbohydrates: 25g | Fiber: 2g | Sugar: 15g

Carrot Cake Protein Balls

These protein balls offer a delicious and portable treat while adhering to a low-FODMAP diet.

Prep Time: 15 minutes || Cook Time: None || Yield: 12-15 balls

INGREDIENTS

- 1 cup gluten-free oats

- 1/2 cup grated carrot

- 1/4 cup peanut butter (low-FODMAP)

- 1/4 cup maple syrup

- 1 tablespoon chia seeds

- 1 teaspoon ground cinnamon

- 1/4 teaspoon ginger

- Pinch of salt

- Optional: chopped walnuts or pecans (low-FODMAP serving size)

INSTRUCTIONS

1. In a food processor, combine oats, grated carrot, peanut butter, maple syrup, chia seeds, cinnamon, ginger, and salt. Pulse until the mixture forms a sticky dough.

2. If the mixture is too dry, add a small amount of water, one tablespoon at a time.

3. If desired, fold in chopped walnuts or pecans.

4. Roll the dough into small balls.

5. Store in the refrigerator for at least 30 minutes to firm up.

NOTES

- For a richer flavor, use a combination of peanut butter and almond butter.

- You can add other spices like nutmeg or cardamom to enhance the carrot cake flavor.

- Store the protein balls in an airtight container in the refrigerator for up to a week.

NUTRITIONAL INFORMATION (approximate per serving):

- Calories: 150 | Protein: 5g | Fat: 8g | Carbohydrates: 18g | Fiber: 3g | Sugar: 5g

Almond & Raspberry Tart

This recipe requires a low-FODMAP tart base, which can be store-bought or homemade.

Prep Time: 30 minutes || **Cook Time:** None || **Yield:** 8 servings

INGREDIENTS

For the filling:

- 1/2 cup almond butter

- 1/4 cup maple syrup

- 1/4 cup coconut cream

- 1 teaspoon vanilla extract

- Pinch of salt

- 1/2 cup fresh raspberries (low-FODMAP serving size)

INSTRUCTIONS

1. In a medium bowl, combine almond butter, maple syrup, coconut cream, vanilla extract, and salt. Beat until smooth and creamy.

2. Gently fold in fresh raspberries.

3. Pour the filling into a prepared low-FODMAP tart base.

4. Refrigerate for at least 2 hours to set.

NOTES

- For a thicker filling, add a small amount of cornstarch or arrowroot flour.

- Adjust sweetness to taste by adding more or less maple syrup.

- Decorate with fresh raspberries or sliced almonds for a festive touch.

- Store leftovers in the refrigerator for up to 3 days.

NUTRITIONAL INFORMATION (approximate per serving):

- Calories: 200 | Protein: 4g | Fat: 12g | Carbohydrates: 15g | Fiber: 2g | Sugar: 10g

Cheesy Mashed Potatoes

A creamy and comforting side dish that's perfect for any meal. This vegan version uses nutritional yeast for a cheesy flavor without dairy.

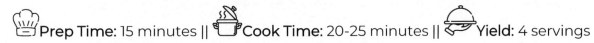

Prep Time: 15 minutes || **Cook Time:** 20-25 minutes || **Yield:** 4 servings

INGREDIENTS

- 2 large russet potatoes, peeled and cubed

- 1/2 cup unsweetened almond milk

- 1/4 cup nutritional yeast

- 2 tablespoons vegan butter (or olive oil)

- 1 clove garlic, minced (optional, for those with mild FODMAP intolerance)

- Salt and pepper to taste

INSTRUCTIONS

1. Place potatoes in a large pot and cover with cold water. Bring to a boil, then reduce heat and simmer until potatoes are tender, about 20-25 minutes.

2. Drain potatoes and return them to the pot.

3. Mash potatoes with a potato masher or ricer until desired consistency.

4. Add almond milk, nutritional yeast, vegan butter (or olive oil), and garlic (if using) to the potatoes. Stir until combined and creamy.

5. Season with salt and pepper to taste. Serve immediately.

NOTES

- For a richer flavor, use full-fat coconut milk instead of almond milk.

- To make the mashed potatoes extra creamy, add a splash of plant-based milk while mashing.

- For a more intense garlic flavor, sauté the garlic in olive oil before adding it to the potatoes.

NUTRITIONAL INFORMATION (approximate per serving):

- Calories: 150 | Protein: 3g | Fat: 5g | Carbohydrates: 25g | Fiber: 2g | Sugar: 1g

PB&J Thumbprint Cookies

A classic childhood treat, reimagined for the low-FODMAP diet. These cookies combine the sweetness of fruit with the creaminess of peanut butter for a satisfying treat. Ensure your peanut butter is low in FODMAPs and choose a low-FODMAP jam for the filling.

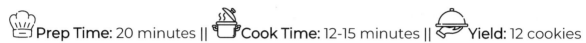 **Prep Time:** 20 minutes || **Cook Time:** 12-15 minutes || **Yield:** 12 cookies

INGREDIENTS

- 1/2 cup creamy peanut butter (low-FODMAP)

- 1/4 cup maple syrup

- 1/4 cup tapioca flour

- 1/4 teaspoon baking powder

- Pinch of salt

- Low-FODMAP jam (e.g., raspberry, strawberry)

INSTRUCTIONS

1. Preheat oven to 350°F (175°C). Line a baking sheet with parchment paper.

2. In a medium bowl, combine peanut butter, maple syrup, tapioca flour, baking powder, and salt. Mix until well combined.

3. Roll the dough into 1-inch balls and place them on the prepared baking sheet.

4. Use your thumb to make a small indentation in the center of each cookie.

5. Fill each indentation with a small amount of low-FODMAP jam.

6. Bake for 12-15 minutes, or until golden brown.

7. Let cool on the baking sheet for a few minutes before transferring to a wire rack to cool completely.

NOTES

- For a nut-free option, use sunflower seed butter or almond butter.

- You can adjust the sweetness by adding more or less maple syrup.

- Store leftovers in an airtight container at room temperature for up to 3 days.

NUTRITIONAL INFORMATION (approximate per serving):

- Calories: 150 | Protein: 4g | Fat: 8g | Carbohydrates: 15g | Fiber: 1g | Sugar: 6g

Veggie Sticks and Hummus

A classic and healthy snack option. This recipe provides a base for customizable veggie sticks and a flavorful hummus dip.

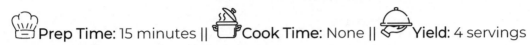 **Prep Time:** 15 minutes || **Cook Time:** None || **Yield:** 4 servings

INGREDIENTS

For the hummus:

- 1 can chickpeas, rinsed and drained

- 3 tablespoons tahini

- 2 tablespoons lemon juice

- 2 tablespoons garlic-infused olive oil

- 1 teaspoon ground cumin

- 1/2 teaspoon smoked paprika

- Salt and pepper to taste

For the veggie sticks:

- 1 large carrot, peeled and sliced

- 1 cucumber, sliced

- 1 red bell pepper, sliced

- Celery sticks (optional, if tolerated)

INSTRUCTIONS

For the hummus:

1. Combine all hummus ingredients in a food processor or blender.

2. Process until smooth and creamy. Add water, a tablespoon at a time, if needed to reach desired consistency. Taste and adjust seasonings as needed.

For the veggie sticks:

1. Wash and prepare your chosen vegetables.

2. Cut vegetables into sticks of desired size and thickness.

NOTES

- For a thicker hummus, add more chickpeas or reduce the amount of olive oil.

- Experiment with different herbs and spices to customize the flavor of your hummus.

- Serve with additional low-FODMAP vegetables like snap peas or sugar snap peas.

NUTRITIONAL INFORMATION (approximate per serving):

- Hummus: Calories 150, Protein 7g, Fat 10g, Carbohydrates 10g, Fiber 4g, Sugar 2g

Sugar-Free Orange Marmalade

This recipe uses a sugar substitute and pectin to achieve a marmalade consistency. Always test the sugar substitute for FODMAP content.

Prep Time: 30 minutes || **Cook Time:** 45-60 minutes || **Yield:** About 3 cups

INGREDIENTS

- 4 large oranges

- 1 cup sugar substitute (low-FODMAP)

- 1 tablespoon liquid pectin

- 1/4 cup water

INSTRUCTIONS

1. Wash the oranges thoroughly.

2. Using a sharp knife, carefully remove the zest from the oranges, avoiding the bitter white pith. Juice the oranges and set aside.

3. Cut the peeled oranges into segments, removing any remaining pith.

4. In a large saucepan, combine orange zest, orange juice, orange segments, sugar substitute, and water.

5. Bring the mixture to a boil, then reduce heat and simmer for 30-45 minutes, or until the mixture thickens. Skim off any foam that rises to the surface.

6. Stir in liquid pectin and cook for an additional 5 minutes, or until the mixture reaches a jam-like consistency. Remove from heat and let cool slightly before transferring to sterilized jars.

7. Seal the jars and store in the refrigerator.

NOTES

- For a thicker marmalade, use a combination of pectin and chia seeds.

- Adjust the sweetness to your taste by adding more or less sugar substitute.

- This marmalade can be used as a spread, topping for yogurt, or as a flavoring for baked goods.

NUTRITIONAL INFORMATION (approximate per serving):

- Calories: 50 | Protein: 1g | Fat: 0g | Carbohydrates: 12g | Fiber: 2g | Sugar: 0g

Dill Veggie Dip with Veggie Sticks

A classic combination of creamy dill dip and crunchy vegetables. This low-FODMAP version is a refreshing and healthy snack option.

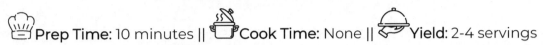 **Prep Time:** 10 minutes || **Cook Time:** None || **Yield:** 2-4 servings

INGREDIENTS

For the dip:

- 1/2 cup vegan mayonnaise (low-FODMAP)

- 1/4 cup plain Greek yogurt (low-FODMAP)

- 2 tablespoons fresh dill, chopped

- 1 tablespoon lemon juice

- 1 teaspoon garlic-infused olive oil (low-FODMAP)

- Salt and pepper to taste

For the veggie sticks:

- 1 carrot, sliced

- 1 cucumber, sliced

- Celery sticks (optional, if tolerated)

- Bell pepper slices (optional)

INSTRUCTIONS

1. In a medium bowl, combine vegan mayonnaise, Greek yogurt, dill, lemon juice, garlic-infused olive oil, salt, and pepper. Stir until well combined.

2. Prepare your chosen vegetables by washing and cutting them into sticks.

3. Serve the dip with the prepared vegetable sticks.

NOTES

- For a thicker dip, use less mayonnaise and more Greek yogurt.

- You can add other herbs like chives or parsley for extra flavor.

- Serve with your favorite low-FODMAP crackers or chips for a more substantial snack.

NUTRITIONAL INFORMATION (approximate per serving):

- Dip: Calories 150, Protein 2g, Fat 12g, Carbohydrates 5g, Fiber 1g, Sugar 1g

- Veggie sticks: Nutritional information varies based on specific vegetables chosen.

Chocolate Chip Breakfast Cookies

These chewy and delicious cookies are packed with wholesome ingredients and perfect for a quick and satisfying breakfast or snack.

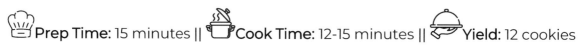 **Prep Time:** 15 minutes || **Cook Time:** 12-15 minutes || **Yield:** 12 cookies

INGREDIENTS

- 1 cup gluten-free oat flour

- 1/2 cup almond flour

- 1/4 teaspoon baking soda

- Pinch of salt

- 1/4 cup maple syrup

- 1/4 cup unsweetened almond milk

- 1 tablespoon flaxseed meal mixed with 3 tablespoons water (flax egg)

- 1 teaspoon vanilla extract

- 1/4 cup vegan chocolate chips (check for low-FODMAP certification)

INSTRUCTIONS

1. Preheat oven to 350°F (175°C). Line a baking sheet with parchment paper.

2. In a large bowl, whisk together oat flour, almond flour, baking soda, and salt.

3. In a separate bowl, whisk together maple syrup, almond milk, flax egg, and vanilla extract.

4. Combine wet ingredients with dry ingredients until just combined. Fold in chocolate chips.

5. Drop by rounded tablespoons onto the prepared baking sheet, leaving space between cookies.

6. Bake for 12-15 minutes, or until golden brown.

7. Let cool on the baking sheet for a few minutes before transferring to a wire rack to cool completely.

NOTES

- For a thicker cookie, chill the dough for 30 minutes before baking.

- Use low-FODMAP certified chocolate chips to ensure they are safe for your diet.

- Store leftovers in an airtight container at room temperature for up to 3 days.

NUTRITIONAL INFORMATION (approximate per serving):

- Calories: 150 | Protein: 3g | Fat: 6g | Carbohydrates: 20g | Fiber: 2g | Sugar: 8g

Eggplant Zucchini Tomato Pasta Sauce

A flavorful and hearty sauce packed with vegetables. This low-FODMAP option is a perfect base for your favorite gluten-free pasta.

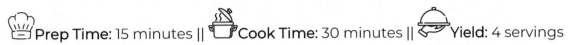

Prep Time: 15 minutes || **Cook Time:** 30 minutes || **Yield:** 4 servings

INGREDIENTS

- 1 tablespoon olive oil

- 1 eggplant, diced

- 1 zucchini, diced

- 1 onion, finely chopped

- 1 clove garlic, minced (optional, for those with mild FODMAP intolerance)

- 1 can (400g) crushed tomatoes

- 1/4 cup tomato paste

- 1/2 teaspoon dried oregano

- 1/4 teaspoon red pepper flakes (optional)

- Salt and pepper to taste

- Fresh basil, for garnish (optional)

INSTRUCTIONS

1. Heat olive oil in a large skillet over medium heat. Add eggplant and zucchini, cook until softened, about 10 minutes.

2. Add onion and garlic (if using), cook until softened, about 5 minutes more.

3. Stir in crushed tomatoes, tomato paste, oregano, and red pepper flakes. Bring to a simmer, reduce heat, and cook for 20-25 minutes, or until thickened.

4. Season with salt and pepper to taste.

5. Serve over your favorite gluten-free pasta. Garnish with fresh basil (optional).

NOTES

- For a richer sauce, roast the eggplant and zucchini before adding them to the pan.

- Adjust the spice level by adding more or less red pepper flakes.

- Serve with additional toppings such as vegan parmesan (low-FODMAP) or pine nuts (check serving size).

NUTRITIONAL INFORMATION (approximate per serving):

- Calories: 200 | Protein: 4g | Fat: 8g | Carbohydrates: 20g | Fiber: 4g | Sugar: 5g

Rice Pudding with Mixed Berry Sauce

A comforting and creamy dessert that's perfect for any occasion. This low-FODMAP version is packed with flavor and is gentle on the digestive system.

Prep Time: 20 minutes + cooling time || **Cook Time:** 30 minutes || **Yield:** 4 servings

INGREDIENTS

For the rice pudding:

- 1/2 cup low-FODMAP rice (such as brown rice or short-grain white rice)

- 2 cups unsweetened almond milk

- 1/4 cup maple syrup

- 1 teaspoon vanilla extract

- Pinch of salt

For the mixed berry sauce:

- 1 cup mixed berries (strawberries, raspberries, blueberries)

- 1 tablespoon cornstarch

- 1 tablespoon water

- 1 tablespoon maple syrup

- 1/4 teaspoon lemon juice

INSTRUCTIONS

For the rice pudding:

1. In a medium saucepan, combine rice, almond milk, maple syrup, vanilla extract, and salt.

2. Bring to a boil, then reduce heat to low and simmer for 25-30 minutes, or until rice is tender and liquid has absorbed.

3. Stir occasionally to prevent sticking.

4. Remove from heat and let cool completely before serving.

For the mixed berry sauce:

1. In a small saucepan, combine mixed berries, cornstarch, water, maple syrup, and lemon juice.

2. Bring to a simmer over medium heat, stirring constantly until thickened.

3. Remove from heat and let cool slightly before serving.

NOTES

- For a thicker rice pudding, use more rice or less almond milk.

- Adjust sweetness to taste by adding more or less maple syrup.

- Serve warm or cold with the mixed berry sauce.

- Store leftovers in the refrigerator for up to 3 days.

NUTRITIONAL INFORMATION (approximate per serving):

- Calories: 200 | Protein: 3g | Fat: 5g | Carbohydrates: 35g | Fiber: 2g | Sugar: 12g

KITCHEN CONVERSIONS

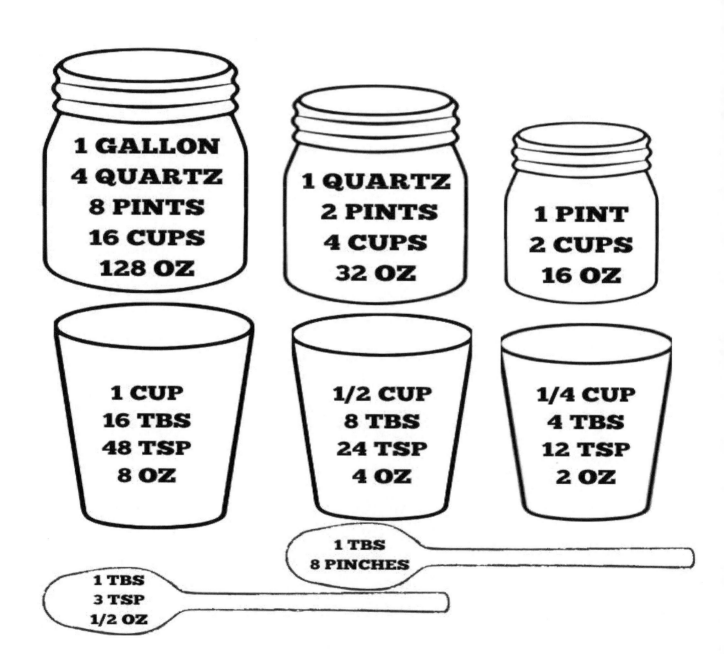

1 GALLON
4 QUARTZ
8 PINTS
16 CUPS
128 OZ

1 QUARTZ
2 PINTS
4 CUPS
32 OZ

1 PINT
2 CUPS
16 OZ

1 CUP
16 TBS
48 TSP
8 OZ

1/2 CUP
8 TBS
24 TSP
4 OZ

1/4 CUP
4 TBS
12 TSP
2 OZ

1 TBS
8 PINCHES

1 TBS
3 TSP
1/2 OZ

Dates

	BREAKFAST	LUNCH	DINNER	SNACKS
MON				
TUE				
WED				
THU				
FRI				
SAT				
SUN				

Shopping list

Dates

_____

	BREAKFAST	LUNCH	DINNER	SNACKS
MON				
TUE				
WED				
THU				
FRI				
SAT				
SUN				

Shopping list

_____   _____   _____

_____   _____   _____

_____   _____   _____

_____   _____   _____

_____   _____   _____

Dates _____

	BREAKFAST	LUNCH	DINNER	SNACKS
MON				
TUE				
WED				
THU				
FRI				
SAT				
SUN				

Shopping list

_____   _____   _____
_____   _____   _____
_____   _____   _____
_____   _____   _____
_____   _____   _____

Dates
_____

	BREAKFAST	LUNCH	DINNER	SNACKS
MON				
TUE				
WED				
THU				
FRI				
SAT				
SUN				

Shopping list

_____ _____ _____
_____ _____ _____
_____ _____ _____
_____ _____ _____
_____ _____ _____

GROCERY LIST

DATE: /   /

DAIRY:
- ○ _____
- ○ _____
- ○ _____
- ○ _____
- ○ _____
- ○ _____
- ○ _____
- ○ _____
- ○ _____
- ○ _____
- ○ _____
- ○ _____

MEAT & SEAFOOD:
- ○ _____
- ○ _____
- ○ _____
- ○ _____
- ○ _____
- ○ _____
- ○ _____
- ○ _____
- ○ _____
- ○ _____
- ○ _____
- ○ _____

FRUITS & VEGGIES:
- ○ _____
- ○ _____
- ○ _____
- ○ _____
- ○ _____
- ○ _____
- ○ _____
- ○ _____

BREAD & CEREAL:
- ○ _____
- ○ _____
- ○ _____
- ○ _____
- ○ _____

OTHERS:
- ○ _____
- ○ _____
- ○ _____
- ○ _____
- ○ _____
- ○ _____
- ○ _____
- ○ _____

FROZEN FOODS:
- ○ _____
- ○ _____
- ○ _____
- ○ _____
- ○ _____

CANNED GOODS:
- ○ _____
- ○ _____
- ○ _____
- ○ _____
- ○ _____

WHAT'S COOKING:
- S
- M
- T
- W
- T
- F
- S

GROCERY LIST

DATE: / /

DAIRY:
- ○ _____
- ○ _____
- ○ _____
- ○ _____
- ○ _____
- ○ _____
- ○ _____
- ○ _____
- ○ _____
- ○ _____
- ○ _____
- ○ _____

MEAT & SEAFOOD:
- ○ _____
- ○ _____
- ○ _____
- ○ _____
- ○ _____
- ○ _____
- ○ _____
- ○ _____
- ○ _____
- ○ _____
- ○ _____
- ○ _____

FRUITS & VEGGIES:
- ○ _____
- ○ _____
- ○ _____
- ○ _____
- ○ _____
- ○ _____
- ○ _____
- ○ _____

BREAD & CEREAL:
- ○ _____
- ○ _____
- ○ _____
- ○ _____
- ○ _____

OTHERS:
- ○ _____
- ○ _____
- ○ _____
- ○ _____
- ○ _____
- ○ _____
- ○ _____

FROZEN FOODS:
- ○ _____
- ○ _____
- ○ _____
- ○ _____
- ○ _____

CANNED GOODS:
- ○ _____
- ○ _____
- ○ _____
- ○ _____
- ○ _____

WHAT'S COOKING:
- S _____
- M _____
- T _____
- W _____
- T _____
- F _____
- S _____

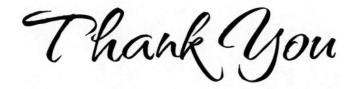

Thank You

Dear Reader,

Thank you for purchasing this cookbook. Creating this cookbook has been a labor of love, and I hope it has inspired you to explore new flavors and techniques in your kitchen. Each recipe has been crafted with care and passion, with the aim to cater to your health and diet requirements.

Your support means the world to me, and I am deeply grateful for your trust in my recipes. As you cook your way through the pages of this book, I hope you find as much joy in making these dishes as I did in creating them.

Jane Garraway

Your Feedback Matters

I would love to hear about your experiences with the recipes in this cookbook. Your honest reviews and feedback are incredibly valuable and help me continue to improve and share the joy of cooking with others. Whether it's a dish that turned out perfectly or one that you think could use some tweaking, your insights are welcomed and appreciated.

Please consider leaving a review on the platform where you purchased this book. Your feedback helps guide future books and ensures that I can continue to provide recipes that resonate with home cooks everywhere.

Thank you once again for your support.

Made in United States
Troutdale, OR
11/02/2024

24370770R00055